INFECTIOUS
DISEASE
REVIEWS

INFECTIOUS DISEASE REVIEWS

Edited by
WILLIAM J. HOLLOWAY, M.D.
Director, Infectious Disease Research Laboratory,
Wilmington Medical Center, Wilmington, Delaware

VOLUME I

7th and 8th Infectious Disease Symposia
Wilmington Medical Center, Delaware

Futura Publishing Company

Published by
Futura Publishing Company Inc.
295 Main Street
Mount Kisco, New York 10549

Printed in the United States of America

Contents

Introduction

The First Annual Infectious Disease Symposium was held in Wilmington, Delaware in 1964 at the instance of E. G. Scott, M.S., who was then Director of Microbiology at the Delaware Hospital (now a division of the Wilmington Medical Center). Mr. Scott recognized the value of such a symposium in the development of the local research effort in infectious diseases. He was joined in his forsightedness by the hospital administrator, R. S. Griffith, who provided financial and technical support. Since that initial meeting the annual Delaware Infectious Disease Symposium has prospered with significant growth in content, scope, attendance, and support. The Delaware Academy of Medicine, the Wilmington Medical Center, and the Delaware Tuberculosis and Health Society cooperate with the pharmaceutical industry to support this outstanding educational event.

Each year authorities in the field of infectious diseases from the United States and abroad participate in formal lectures, round table presentations, and informal discussion periods. Participants are invited to present material on any aspect of infectious diseases and this freedom results in a diversity of topics increasing the range of appeal to our potential audience.

In the past few years, clinical investigators have been invited to present their experience with new antimicrobial agents, new uses for older antibiotics, or new methods of diagnosis of infections. Local investigators working in our Infectious Disease Research Program have contributed such material to the Symposium.

The sponsors of the Delaware Infectious Disease Symposium appreciate the opportunity to hear outstanding scientists exchange ideas and propagate controversies. Therefore, since 1965 these symposia have been taped and the proceedings made available to local physicians and paramedical personnel unable to attend the meetings. By 1970, it was recognized that publication of the papers presented would offer this information to a larger group of clinicians and scientists. The Delaware Medical Journal graciously agreed to print papers submitted from the Seventh and Eighth Annual Infectious Disease Symposia in its November, 1970 and November, 1971 issues.

During the past two years many friends have called it to our attention that although The Delaware Medical Journal is a revered publication with a long history of serving the medical profession of Delaware, it does not enjoy a wide circulation. This deprives many potential readers the opportunity of reviewing the papers presented at this annual infectious disease meeting. The editor of The Delaware Medical Journal has magnanimously given us permission to publish in a single volume the papers from the Seventh and Eighth Infectious Disease Symposia. Our plan for the Ninth Annual Infectious Disease Symposium (held in May, 1972) and future symposia is to publish each year's proceedings as a single volume.

In this volume covering the Seventh and Eighth Symposia, the reader's attention is called to two articles dealing with the undesirable side effects of antibiotics both written by authorities in this field. A review of related interest is Dr. Maxwell Finland's excellent summary of the controversial subject of antibiotic combinations.

Authoritative summaries of hepatic abscess, anaerobic infections, tuberculosis, fungal infections, and respiratory viral infections enhance the value of this volume.

Clinicians interested in the vagaries of urinary tract infections will benefit from four articles directed to the diagnosis and localization of such infections. In addition, five articles present experience with new antibacterial agents in the treatment of urinary tract infections. Several papers are devoted to the epidemiology, diagnosis, and treatment of gonorrhea.

The novice and the expert in infectious disease will enjoy the discourse on the approach to fever of unknown origin.

The Wilmington Symposium attracts a wide range of physicians and scientists, so it is necessary that the program be designed to interest a diverse group. The broad coverage afforded herein makes this volume a valuable addition to the library of those whose interests lie in this direction.

ADVERSE EFFECTS OF ANTIBACTERIAL AGENTS

• Proper antibiotic usage requires familiarity with the pharmacology and toxicology of these agents. Antibiotic induced diseases are becoming more prevalent and should be recognized by the practicing physician.

WILLIAM BRUMFITT, M.D., Ph.D.,
M.R.C.P., F.R.C. Path.

In Britain antibiotics are the most widely used drugs obtained on a doctor's prescription. It is a tribute to the safety of these drugs that they are used so widely with minimum toxic effects. It is also true to say that many of the toxic reactions which have been reported with the commonly used antibiotics have resulted from their unnecessary use or gross error in dosage. Overdosage may be absolute, but sometimes the overdosage is relative. For example, a defect in excretion due to impaired renal function can cause accumulation to a toxic level even when the drug is given in a dose well below that which is normally recommended. Some of the complications which have been described are rare but have been highlighted because they provide a means of investigating other medical disciplines. For instance, penicillin-induced hemolytic anemia, or hemolytic anemia that follows the use of certain antimicrobials when there is a glucose 6-phosphate dehydrogenase deficiency, may be of special interest to hematologists, and hence this subject has been widely reported in the medical literature. Some of these special conditions will be dealt with in more detail later.

The complications related to antimicrobial therapy can be divided into pharmacological and biological, and Table I gives examples of the pharmacological complications. Absolute

Dr. Brumfitt, Ph.D., M.C.R.P., F.R.C. Path., is Consultant Clinical Pathologist, Edgware General Hospital; Consultant Bacteriologist, St. Mary's Hospital, London, W. 2; and Senior Lecturer in Bacteriology at the University of London.

overdosage usually results from an error in prescribing, but occasionally deliberate overdosage is necessary to eradicate infection as a lifesaving measure. Relative overdosage occurs most often in association with renal failure. In the presence of impaired renal function certain drugs, such as the aminoglycosides, nitrofurans and amphotericin B, are particularly dangerous and frequently produce serious toxicity. Similarly, certain drugs are dangerous in hepatic failure, where there are enzyme defects, immaturity of the detoxicating mechanisms or, in certain circumstances, drug interactions.

An example of relative overdosage due to an enzyme deficiency is illustrated in Figure 1. The simplified diagram attempts to show the mechanism of hemolytic anemia due to glucose 6-phosphate dehydrogenase deficiency. Sulfonamides, nitrofurans and nalidixic acid are only some examples of antimicrobial agents which can precipitate a hemolytic anemia in patients with this enzyme deficiency. The figure shows how sulfonamide normally combines with hemoglobin to produce the oxidized compound methemoglobin. However, this reaction is normally reversed by methemoglobin reductase which depends on the pentose shunt producing TPNH. The TPNH production is, in turn, dependent upon glucose 6-phosphate being converted to 6-phosphogluconate for which the enzyme glucose 6-phosphate dehydrogenase (G-6-PD) is required. If methemoglobin is not reduced back

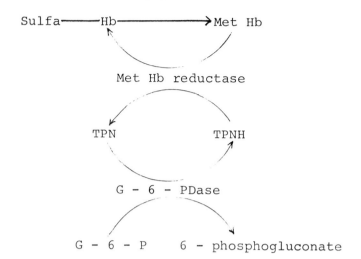

FIGURE 1

Diagram to illustrate the way in which sulfonamide may cause hemolytic anemia in patients with glucose - 6 - phosphate dehydrogenase deficiency.

to oxyhemoglobin, then the denatured hemoglobin results in the characteristic Heinz body anemia, which is associated with intravascular hemolysis and hemoglobinuria.

From the medical literature it might be supposed that this condition is common in those races where deficiency of G-6-PD is often found. However, not all workers agree that hemolytic anemia following the administration of these drugs is common, even in populations where the enzyme deficiency has been shown to be severe. Furthermore, where a deficiency is present in the Negro, and hemolytic anemia occurs, it is less severe because only mature red cells are deficient in the enzyme, whereas newly formed red cells and reticulocytes contain the enzyme in normal amounts. Thus, only the *mature* red cells are destroyed, and severe anemia does not result.

In Asiatics, however, all red cells may be deficient, and the resulting hemolytic anemia can, therefore, be of great severity. Nevertheless, it is interesting that in some countries where this deficiency is common and sulfonamides are withheld for the treatment of infection, diabetic patients are treated with the sulfonylurea group of oral antidiabetics, apparently with little trouble.

The biological complications (Table II) are no less important. For example, following administration of chemotherapeutic substances by mouth, change in bowel flora or direct action of these substances on the bowel wall can give rise to complications varying in severity from pseudo-membranous enterocolitis to the less serious, but nevertheless highly inconvenient, complication of diarrhea. Other well known biological effects include suppression of antibody synthesis, liberation of toxic components from microorganisms, specifically seen in the Jarisch-Herxheimer reaction, and, perhaps more remotely, the masking of infections by an agent which is only partially active. Some of these adverse reactions of chemotherapeutic agents will be dealt with later in detail. Before going on to these, however, it is worth emphasizing that a very important complication of chemotherapy is the use of an ineffective drug. This may be due to incorrect prescribing, but other causes, such as failure to appreciate the instability of some antibiotics when made in solution, are important. This especially causes problems when an unstable antibiotic is added to an intravenous infusion fluid. Difficulties also arise when compounds require special conditions for their action; for instance, hexamine

4

Overdosage	
Accidental	
Deliberate (lifesaving)	
Relative overdosage	
Renal failure	Aminoglycosides, Nitrofurans
Hepatic failure	Tetracyclines
Enzyme defects	Nitrofurans, Sulfonamides
Immaturity	Chloramphenicol in neonates
Drug interactions	
	Aminoglycosides and muscle relaxants

TABLE I

ANTIBIOTIC THERAPY
Pharmacological
Complications
(Dose Related and Specific)

mandelate is only active in the urine when the pH is lowered to 5 or below. It is insufficiently appreciated that irregular absorption from the alimentary canal occurs with many commonly used antibiotics. For example, failure to give instructions about taking antibiotics in relation to food can, in some cases, lead to poor absorption, while in sick people absorption of antibiotics is known to be irregular.

Finally, an incorrect bacteriological diagnosis or failure of a clinician to appreciate a bacteriologist's report in relation to the specific infection with which he is dealing, can result in errors of treatment. I have seen nitrofurantoin used for the treatment of a pulmonary staphylococcal infection on the basis of a laboratory report, although it is well known that this substance does not produce an effective concentration of antibacterial substance at any site other than the urinary tract.

The Sulfonamides

In Table III some of the unwanted effects of sulfonamides are listed. These vary from nausea to polyarteritis nodosa. The latter condition rarely follows the use of sulfonamides, and the causal role of these compounds is not established definitely.

Jaundice has been reported following sulfonamide administration and can be of two varieties. In infants whose mothers have received sulfonamides late in pregnancy, it is theoretically possible that the sulfonamide crossing the placenta will compete with bilirubin for conjugation with glucuronic acid.[1,2]

However, this complication of sulfonamides is apparently a theoretical one, for Adamsons and Joelsson[3] claim that it is unlikely that enough sulfonamide can cross the placenta to conjugate with sufficient binding sites to cause serious hyperbilirubinemia. It is therefore improbable that jaundice will result from this cause, and the evidence that such therapy has ever been the cause of kernicterus is unproven. Nevertheless, it would probably be advisable to avoid sulfonamide in the later stages of pregnancy if there is rhesus incompatibility, or in neonates where delivery has been premature.

Sulfonamides have also been reported to cause hepatocellular jaundice. A raised transaminase with eosinophilia is characteristic of the condition, and liver biopsy shows multiple focal areas of cell necrosis, prominent bile casts and other evidence of intrahepatic cholestasis. It is postulated that the mechanism is acquired hypersensitivity.[4] The actual number of patients reported during the last 30 years, which includes a period of about ten years when sulfonamides were the only antibacterial agents available, is 108. The jaundice resolves when the sulfonamide is withdrawn, no deaths have been recorded, and there is no doubt that the danger of sulfonamide in causing such an hepatic lesion is substantially less than with some other widely used drugs, such as chlorpromazine.

Hemopoietic disturbances have also been reported, and in particular depression of marrow function. However, in contrast to that

5

TABLE II

ANTIBIOTIC THERAPY

Biological Complications

Change in bacterial flora
    Pseudomembranous enterocolitis
    Suppression of Vitamin K synthesis
Suppression of antibody synthesis
    Typhus and typhoid
Liberation of toxic components from
microorganisms
    Jarisch-Herxheimer reaction
Masking of infections by a partially active
agent
    S.B.E.   Inadequate or bacteriostatic dose

caused by chloramphenicol, recovery usually occurs when the sulfonamide is withdrawn.

Renal crystalluria was at one time an important problem following administration of sulfonamides, but, with the more recently developed derivatives, this complication is rare, provided that precautions to maintain an adequate urine flow are taken.

Finally, and perhaps most important, is the question of skin rash and in particular the Stevens-Johnson syndrome. (Table III) Of course, the report of Stevens and Johnson was made in 1922, long before sulfonamides were available, but later sulfonamides were incriminated and the long-acting derivatives have been said to be particularly dangerous[5] although, since the original report, Beveridge[6] has seen no further cases. The Federal Drug Administration reported 116 cases and 20 deaths, but this must be viewed in a proper perspective for the frequency seems to be one to two cases per million daily doses, and the Norwegian worker Wereide[7] has calculated that the risk of developing this syndrome is of the order of one patient per metric ton (thousand kilograms) administered.

It is salutary to note that a number of patients who have developed the Stevens-Johnson syndrome following the administration of sulfonamide have been given the drug for dubious reasons, such as prophylaxis during an attack of measles or for undiagnosed fever. This necessarily raises the question as to whether the sulfonamide was always the true or sole etiological agent or whether the underlying illness should also be implicated. It is interesting that sulfonamides have been used widely for the prophylaxis of rheumatic fever without causing this complication.

Nevertheless, the most important toxic effect of sulfonamides is in relation to a wide range of skin lesions due to hypersensitivity reactions. Table III shows that these can range from transient localized rash to the typical diffuse maculo-erythematous rash, with or without urticaria, and in the more severe forms this may become confluent. As already indicated, the more serious complications, such as the Stevens-Johnson syndrome and Lyell's syndrome, are rare. It is important to appreciate that the varieties of skin hypersensitivity shown in Table III represent a continuous spectrum of increasing severity, rather than being separate entities, although it is true that distinct and unrelated manifestations of sulfonamide hypersensitivity, such as erythema nodosum, also occur.

Two final points arise, firstly that sulfonamide toxicity varies from compound to compound (Table IV) and the statement that long acting sulfonamides are more likely to cause severe skin manifestations is not substantiated in the literature.[8] In this context it is not widely appreciated that some of the standard forms of sulfonamide (for example, sulfadiazine, half life 18 hours) have not been incriminated with the Stevens-Johnson syndrome, though they are in fact long acting. Secondly, it is worth remembering that the antidiabetic sulfonylureas are closely related chemically to the antibacterial sulfonamides, and that some of these, such as chlorpropamide (half life 36 hours) are also long acting. Table V compares the toxic effects of carbutamide, which has both an antibacterial and antidiabetic action, with tolbutamide, which has only an antidiabetic action. The latter has been described as the safest drug since coffee, without an outcry from the medical profession, although it can be seen that these sulfonylureas cause side effects similar to those found with sulfonamides used for the treatment of infection.

Nausea
Polyarteritis nodosa
Jaundice   —Neonatal (with kernicterus)
                     Hepatocellular in adults

Renal crystalluria
Hemopoietic disturbances
Dermatological   —Hypersensitivity
   Rash   — local, diffuse, confluent maculo-erythematous
          (sometimes with urticaria)

  Erythema multiforme
  Lyell's syndrome
  Stevens- Johnson syndrome

     Frequency 1-2 cases/10^6 daily doses
             116 cases (79 under 15 years)
              20 deaths

TABLE III

SOME IMPORTANT UNWANTED EFFECTS RESULTING FROM ADMINISTRATION OF THE SULFONAMIDES

It has been said that the long-acting sulfonamides are dangerous because the persistence of the rash will be related to the time that the drug is retained in the body. However, I have personally seen an example of a sulfonamide rash following the use of the ultra-long acting compound sulfadoxine which disappeared within half an hour in spite of sustained levels of the compound in the serum.[9]

The Penicillins

It is interesting to speculate whether penicillin would have been put on the market if animal toxicity tests had been carried out. Administration to the guinea pig results in coliform invasion of the blood stream from the gut, which is fatal in a few days. Of course, this effect is not seen in the human, where toxicity is rare. Trouble only arises when massive parenteral doses are given, so that penicillin crosses the blood brain barrier in sufficient concentration to cause damage or when an excessive dosage is given by the intrathecal

TABLE IV

The Toxicity of Three Different Sulfonamides in Relation to Nausea, Vomiting, Headache, Dizziness, Drug Fever and Sensitization

Sulfafurazole	1%
Sulfadiazine	6%
Sulfathiazole	18%

route. In fact, toxicity in the human associated with large doses of penicillin is more likely to result from hyperkalemia due to the use of the potassium salt, or from hypokalemia resulting from use of the sodium salt rather than from the penicillin itself.

When using penicillin for the treatment of syphilis, it is important to remember the Herxheimer reaction, which results from release of a specific toxic substance at the site of the spirochetal invasion. In early syphilis 50% of patients given penicillin develop an influenza-like illness, with fever, whereas in late syphilis collapse and death may occur. The latter is due either to local effects, such as occlusion of the coronary arteries, when there is an associated syphilitic aortitis, or to a diffuse anaphylactoid reaction.

At the present time much attention is being focused on the problem of hypersensitivity to the penicillins because such reactions are by no means uncommon. However, reports of the actual incidence of hypersensitivity vary from author to author, and there is also considerable confusion about the etiology of this condition. Hypersensitivity may result from large molecular contaminants, either from the amidase used to remove the side chain in the semi-synthetic synthesis of the new penicillins or from the actual mold (*P. chrysogenum*) used in penicillin production. This theory goes some way to explaining why penicillin by

7

TABLE V

Toxic Effects of the Antidiabetic
Sulfonylureas

	Carbutamide	Tolbutamide
No. Studied	3,936	3,582
Side effects	5.44%	2.46%
Skin allergy	3.6%	0.8%
G.I. disturbance	1.6%	1.6%
Drug fever	0.12%	0.03%
Blood dyscrasia	0.12%	0.03%

injection is more likely to produce hypersensitivity than penicillin administered by the oral route, since many of the large molecular contaminants would be either destroyed or not absorbed from the alimentary canal. Alternatively, hypersensitivity can result from degradation products of penicillin, especially the penicilloyl derivatives. These may be formed *in vitro* and are therefore related to the concentration, temperature and time of storage of the penicillin *in vitro*, but they may also be formed *in vivo*. At the present time there is controversy as to whether the large molecular contaminants or degradation products are more important in causing skin hypersensitivity. A recent report from the United States of side effects in hospitals where different brands of ampicillin were used is most interesting, for the incidence of hypersensitivity was significantly different.[10] In this investigation it was noted that the incidence was related to the suppliers of the ampicillin, suggesting, of course, that different products vary in their ability to cause reactions. These observations clearly deserve further investigation.

Finally, it should be noted that the penicillin monomer tends to undergo polymerization when in solution *(in vitro* and *in vivo)* following opening of the β-lactam ring, which then links covalently with other similar molecules. The resulting high molecular weight polymer acts as a haptene and by combination with preformed antibody can then cause hypersensitivity reactions. The actual mechanism of hypersensitivity is therefore obscure but can be divided broadly into at least three

different varieties, large molecular weight contaminants, penicillanic acid or other penicilloyl derivatives and high molecular weight polymers.

The type of hypersensitivity reaction also varies. Immediate profound shock may occur and is associated with reaginic antibodies of the IgE class which bind rapidly to receptor sites, but serum sickness and rashes (usually maculopapular) are associated with IgG antibody. Previous exposure to penicillin, either by therapy or by hidden contact with products such as milk, always seems to have occurred in patients who develop hypersensitivity reactions. (The few patients who reacted to penicillin when it was first introduced in 1944 may well have been allergic to the various contaminants present in the suspending agent.) Sensitization may also have been due to contamination of syringes, although this will be unusual in the future because of the introduction of disposable products, but contamination of articles with penicillin in the hospital ward can sometimes be important in sensitization.

The diagnosis of penicillin allergy is far from easy, and it must be remembered that some of the direct tests may themselves precipitate a severe reaction. For this reason, attempts have been made to develop indirect methods. The hemagglutination test, where red cells together with an appropriate antigen are incubated with the patient's serum to see whether agglutination occurs,[11] has not proved to be useful. The basophile degranulation test,[12] in which the antigen and the patient's serum are incubated with basophiles which are then examined for degranulation, has been used by many investigators. Hypersensitivity was claimed to be present when degranulation occurred, but this test has not been found to be reliable in practice. Yet another *in vitro* test is the use of lymphocyte culture to see whether incubation with the specific antigen results in their conversion to blast-forms. In the hands of some workers the test has proved to be successful in predicting allergy[13] whereas others have expressed serious reservations about the value of the test.[14]

Another approach to the diagnosis of allergy is by cutaneous testing, using either the

Diagnosis	Cephaloridine dosage in gm per day			Total Cases
	>6	6 for 5 days	<6	
S.B.E.	4	3	3	10
Septicemia		2		2
Kidney infections	2	1	5	8
Lung infections	2	1	4	7
Others	5	1	3	9
Total Cases	13	8	15	36

TABLE VI

CEPHALORIDINE
NEPHROTOXICITY

penicillin itself or, more usually, the penicilloyl derivatives. It is claimed that the penicilloyl polylysine derivative gives more accurate results than the parent penicillin compound and, at the same time, is much less likely to produce a severe reaction.[15] However, not all workers agree that this test is a reliable one, and some have found the test to be positive in only 60% of patients who are sensitive to penicillin. There is also at least one report[16] of this test causing cutaneous manifestations of penicillin hypersensitivity. Whenever cutaneous tests are being carried out, it is wise to have a syringe containing adrenaline available to deal with any emergency that may arise. Finally, the possibility of using passive transfer experiments with serum from hypersensitive patients is, at present, being explored, using the monkey and rabbit.

The rash following the use of penicillin is highly characteristic and may occur any time between one hour and 30 days. However, following the first administration of a penicillin, it is usually seen between the fifth and ninth day of treatment, but on the second and subsequent occasions the onset may be much more rapid. A most interesting observation is that of Pullen and his colleagues in Edinburgh,[17] who found that ampicillin given for the treatment of glandular fever (an illness, incidentally, for which there is usually no indication for chemotherapy) increases the risk of rash greatly. In fact, the use of ampicillin in this condition may be a better diagnostic test for the disease than the Paul-Bunnell because the incidence of rash following the use of ampicillin in glandular fever has

been reported to be as high as 80%. Benzyl penicillin also causes similar hypersensitivity reactions but in only 40% of patients.[18] The rash resulting from the administration of ampicillin in glandular fever is characteristic of penicillin hypersensitivity and is often very severe. The possibility that the abnormal protein produced in glandular fever combines with the ampicillin haptene to form a complete antigen must be considered.

A reaction confined to the use of methicillin is the syndrome of neutropenia and nephropathy.

The cephalosporins are, of course, closely related to the penicillins, and these compounds can themselves produce a rash very similar, if not identical, to that caused by penicillin. The important question as to whether there is cross-reactivity with the penicillins is at present being actively investigated. In the meantime, it would seem to be reasonable to recommend that patients known to be sensitive to penicillin should not be given cephalosporins if an alternative antibiotic is available.

Cephalosporin Nephrotoxicity

A complication of cephalosporin therapy which seems restricted to cephaloridine is that of nephrotoxicity. This complication has not been reported with either cephalothin or cephalexin. It is therefore pertinent to examine the differences between the cephalosporins. When cephaloridine and cephalothin are compared, it is apparent that cephaloridine differs from cephalothin in not being metabolized, in being painless on injection, and

9

in giving higher and more sustained blood levels. It is also excreted by the glomeruli, and this may be related to the risk of renal toxicity. It is important to note that the risk of nephrotoxicity with cephaloridine is enhanced if certain diuretics (particularly furosemide) are given at the same time. The interesting possibility that the toxicity is associated with renin production must be considered in view of the recent report by Brown and his colleagues.[19]

The lesion produced following cephaloridine nephrotoxicity is an acute tubular necrosis, which particularly affects the proximal tubule. Following withdrawal of the drug, the lesion is reversible. Table VI shows details of 36 patients who developed this complication,[20] and it can be seen that it is very much more likely to occur when the dosage of cephaloridine is in excess of 6 gm daily.

Although 15 cases have been observed with doses of less than 6 gm, it must be appreciated that doses of this order are very much more commonly administered than doses exceeding 6 gm daily. Furthermore, the presence of renal failure in various degrees enhances the risk of the complication, and it is important to note that ten of the 36 cases were associated with bacterial endocarditis, and a further ten were suffering from septicemia or renal infection.

Since the renal lesion is reversible, peritoneal or hemodialysis must be considered for patients who develop renal failure due to nephrotoxicity following cephaloridine therapy.

The Aminoglycosides

Streptomycin This substance may cause pain on injection, and other immediate effects include parasthesiae around the mouth, vertigo and ataxia. However, the most important toxic effect is damage to the eighth nerve, and during short-term therapy this complication can nearly always be attributed to a dose which gives an excessively high blood level. It should be appreciated that a single very large dose can cause nerve damage, since once the substance reaches the endolymph, there will be a considerable lag period before it is eliminated. Animal experiments have localized the effect of the aminoglycosides to the sensory epithelia of the labyrinth.

Eighth nerve damage is also related to the duration of therapy, and in this context it is important to remember that older patients, and particularly those over the age of 50, not only are more likely to develop eighth nerve damage but also that, when this damage does occur, such patients are less well able to compensate. Care is also necessary when treating pregnant women because placental transfer of the streptomycin can occur causing damage to the eighth nerve of the fetus.

Other important toxic effects of streptomycin include hypersensitivity, which leads to a characteristic drug rash, with or without fever. This complication occurs in five per cent of patients given the drug and, although usually trivial, can be severe on occasion, and even fatal exfoliative dermatitis may develop. The drug rash may also be associated with lymphadenopathy.

Finally, it must be remembered that where streptomycin is administered in combination with other substances causing neuromuscular blockade, an additive or synergistic reaction may occur because of the action of streptomycin in reducing the sensitivity of the post-junctional end-plate membrane to the depolarizing effect of acetyl-choline. Thus, the use of streptomycin in combination with muscle relaxant drugs is best avoided, including the use of intraperitoneal streptomycin at operation.

Kanamycin and Gentamicin The aminoglycosides, kanamycin and gentamicin, are valuable in the treatment of bacteremia with hypotension. In such patients renal excretion may be impaired, and conventional dosage can therefore lead to high blood levels. Labyrinthine function may be affected, and this can become apparent both during therapy and between one and fourteen days after treatment. It is my practice to carry out daily visits on patients confined to bed and ask them to sit up and tell me whether they notice anything wrong. If they complain of symptoms such as imbalance, suggesting labyrinthine damage, I withdraw the drug immediately unless its continued use is essential as a lifesaving measure. It should be emphasized that such clinical observations are an indication for stopping these substances, even when blood levels are within normal limits. Unfortunately, disturbance of vestibular function may not be noticed until the patient becomes ambulant, when the course of treatment has been completed.

Effects on the eighth nerve are unusual if the peak kanamycin blood levels are kept below 20 μg/ml and gentamicin below 10 μg/ml, but it must be remembered that the administration of one excessive dose of either of these antibiotics can result in damage to the labyrinth due to spill over into the endolymph. Since it is impossible to obtain serum for assay of antibiotic level after each dose, the clinician may be unaware that this mishap has occurred, and this may explain occasional examples of toxicity where blood levels have been apparently satisfactory.

The Tetracyclines

Tetracyline is interesting in that cutaneous hypersensitivity is unusual, and when it does occur, it is often associated with certain long-acting compounds, notably demethylchlortetracycline, which can cause photosensitization following prolonged exposure to sunlight. Well-known but serious side effects of tetracycline are nausea, vomiting and diarrhea. The diarrhea may be mild, but it can also be severe and protracted. It is not necessarily dose related, and even after a small dose given for a short duration, diarrhea may continue for several weeks. The evidence that the tetracyclines produce their effects by allowing enhanced growth of *Candida sp.* is widely quoted, but unimpressive.[21] Unlike the penicillin group of drugs, this compound is not broken down in the intestinal canal, and following oral administration, analysis of feces shows levels in excess of 1 mg/gm. Very rarely the administration of tetracycline can precipitate a condition indistinguishable from ulcerative colitis, but the question of whether these patients were particularly liable to develop this condition must be considered. Another complication which has been observed following the administration of tetracycline is pseudomembranous enterocolitis, usually due to antibiotic resistant *Staphylococcus pyogenes*. This condition most often follows operative procedures on the alimentary canal.

That tetracycline can cause staining of teeth due to the chelating action of the tetracyclines seems to be beyond doubt. Staining occurs during calcification of the teeth; thus staining of deciduous teeth usually follows administration of tetracycline to the pregnant female after the fifth month of pregnancy. In the same way, staining of the permanent dentition can occur if tetracycline is given between six months and four years of age. The risk of producing this complication by tetracycline therapy at these times is not known, for there is little information about the incidence in relation to the amount or number of courses of tetracycline given.

Liver damage can result from tetracyclines, especially following intravenous administration, and fatty change and atrophy during pregnancy may be followed by death. The suggestion has been made that the liver damage may be due to degenerate forms of tetracycline (toxic epimers). Further information on this point would be useful in view of the established value of tetracycline in the treatment of *Bacteroides spp.* septicemia, a condition which is now being diagnosed more frequently.

Chloramphenicol

The toxicity of this drug is a very controversial subject. Chloramphenicol is an ana-

---

TABLE VII

Unwanted Effects Following the
Administration of Nitrofurantoin

G.I. Tract	Nausea and vomiting
Allergic	Anaphylaxis
Reactions	Severe asthma
	Pulmonary edema, pleural effusion, eosinophilia
Anemia	Megaloblastic
	Haemolytic G-6-PD deficiency
Skin	Vesicular and morbiliform
Pulmonary infiltration	
Peripheral neuropathy	

11

TABLE VIII

SIDE EFFECTS OF TRIMETHOPRIM-
SULFAMETHOXAZOLE AND PLACEBO

	Active Treatment	Placebo
Number studied	120	66
Vomiting	3	2
Dizziness	2	0
Sore tongue	1	0
Abdominal pain	1	0
Heartburn	0	1
Skin rash	1	0

logue of phenylalanine and binds specifically to the 50S subunit of bacterial ribosomes. The precise locus of its action has not yet been conclusively established, but it is likely that it inhibits the ribosome enzyme responsible for peptide bond formation. Its action, therefore, is to inhibit protein synthesis by blocking the growth of the peptide chain.

In higher microorganisms (yeasts and fungi) and in mammalian cells the site of action has been observed to be on the mitochondria, and its effect on such cells may be related to mitochondrial degeneration which would interfere with respiratory processes.

In animals it has been observed that chloramphenicol can inhibit reticulocytosis in rabbits made acutely anemic, inhibit antibody response and delay rejection of skin grafts. It has also been observed that in patients suffering from pernicious anemia administration of chloramphenicol, together with vitamin B_{12}, delays the reticulocyte response.

Toxicity of chloramphenicol in a newborn child is beyond doubt, and the gray syndrome is well known. Infants given doses of 100-160 mg/kg body weight develop vomiting, refusal to suck and abdominal distention after two or three days, and this is succeeded by flaccidity and ashen color, hypothermia, collapse and finally death.

In the adult, mild gastrointestinal side effects have been observed, but the most important and controversial question is that related to marrow aplasia. In 1963 the American Medical Association reported that of 674 patients developing marrow aplasia, 299 were chloramphenicol induced. Furthermore, marrow aplasia resulting from chloramphenicol tends to be irreversible and results in the death of the patient. However, two points must be borne in mind. First, individual workers report that very large doses have been given without toxicity, and others have observed thousands of patients treated with chloramphenicol without a single instance of marrow depression. Second, chloramphenicol is widely used in certain countries, notably Germany, Italy, and Spain, and a recent report from Israel[22] has shown that not a single case of marrow aplasia has been found after the use of chloramphenicol in thousands of cases.

A final point about chloramphenicol is that the original toxicity tests in animals gave a satisfactory result, and no toxicity was reported, a very salutary finding.

Erythromycin

All varieties of erythromycin can cause diarrhea, nausea and vomiting of varying severity. An important question is whether the estolate, which has the advantage of being better absorbed and therefore giving higher blood levels, is, nevertheless, contra-indicated because of its toxicity. The estolate derivative has been found to cause intrahepatic cholestasis and liver cell necrosis, although there have been no deaths and recovery is complete when the drug is withdrawn. As in the case of other antibiotics, the risk is by no means clear. Robinson[23] found an incidence of hepatitis in 12% of patients receiving therapy with the estolate derivative for more than 14 days, whereas Kohlstaedt[24] in a survey could find only 33 patients suffering from intrahepatic cholestasis following the administration of 15 million doses.

The Nitrofurans

The nitrofurans are somewhat underinvestigated, for they are potentially important chemotherapeutic substances and bacterial resistance does not develop readily. Nausea and vomiting following their administration are well-known, but a number of other toxic side effects have been reported, and these are summarized in Table VII. None of the

FIGURE 2

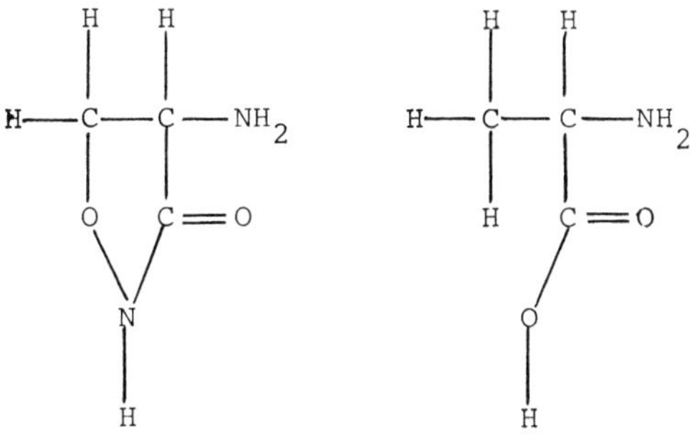

D - cycloserine   D - alanine

---

latter complications are common, but the finding of peripheral neuropathy following the administration of nitrofurantoin in renal failure is of great importance. The drug should not be given in the presence of a raised blood urea, and even tests on normal people by electromyography have shown that abnormal results can be detected, even in patients with normal renal function.

Nalidixic Acid

Again, this drug may cause nausea and diarrhea in 8%, although other side effects are unusual. It is important to remember to advise patients taking nalidixic acid not to expose themselves to the sun for prolonged periods, because of the danger of photosensitization. Visual disturbances with fortification spectra and flashing lights also occur, following the administration of this substance. Although alarming to the patient, these effects stop on withdrawal of the drug. Other effects of therapy rarely seen are vertigo, headache, mental changes, fever with eosinophilia, mild rashes with urticaria and respiratory depression (if respiratory insufficiency is present).

Cycloserine

This is a most interesting drug from the academic point of view. D-alanine is not used in human protein metabolism, and, as cycloserine is an analogue of this amino acid (Figure 2) it might be expected to be of low toxicity.

The action of d-cycloserine is interesting since it causes an accumulation in the cell of a muramic acid residue lacking in the terminal amino-groups. This is because both alanine racemase and d-alanyl-d-alanine synthetase are competitively inhibited by d-cycloserine. D-cycloserine has an affinity for the binding site on alanine racemase which is one hundred times greater than for the natural substrate, so that accumulation of muramic acid residues lacking in the terminal amino-groups on the oligopeptide side chain occurs.

D-cycloserine toxicity is well known and may occur if the blood level exceeds 30 μg/ml. The most important toxic effect is on the central nervous system, and headaches, speech changes, dizziness, convulsions and coma may occur. Psychiatric disturbances ranging from mild changes to psychosis have been reported.

Trimethoprim

The newly introduced drug trimethoprim might be suspected of being toxic in view of its effect on dihydrofolate reductase, the enzyme responsible for the conversion of folic acid to folinic acid. (Figure 3) The lack of toxicity is related to the great difference between the affinity of trimethoprim for the human dihydrofolate reductase, which is extremely low, and its very high affinity for the equivalent bacterial enzyme. The modification to a molecule so as to exhibit differential toxicity is, of course, in keeping, with the approach to chemotherapy advocated by Ehrlich. In considering toxic effects of this drug, we studied the side effects on pregnant women receiving both sulfamethoxazole-trimethoprim combination, and a placebo. It was interesting to find that the number of patients suffering side effects was very similar in the two groups (Table VIII), which emphasizes the importance of using controls in toxicity studies where effects are subjective. However, the potentially serious effects of trimethoprim are, first, the possibility of its causing folate deficiency and thus interfering with hemopoiesis and, second, the relationship to fetal abnormality, since this has been reported in animals. Regarding the effect on hemopoiesis, changes might be expected in the marrow and peripheral granulocytes, red cells and platelets. In investigating such changes it is likely that the most valuable test would be an esti-

13

FIGURE 3

SITES OF ACTION OF SULFONAMIDE AND TRIMETHOPRIM.

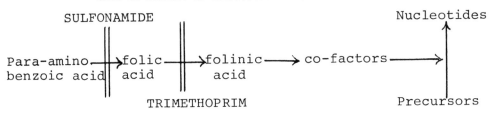

mation of dihydrofolate reductase in either the marrow or peripheral leucocytes before and after treatment. Such work is currently in progress.

Another possible toxic effect of trimethoprim is in the production of fetal abnormalities, since this has been reported in animals.[25] However, we have carried out a follow-up of infants born to mothers treated with trimethoprim and found no evidence of an increased incidence of abnormality.[26]

In relation to teratogenicity caused by treating pregnant women with urinary infections it must be noted that, even if an antimicrobial was shown to cause fetal abnormalities, banning it in pregnancy *only* makes little contribution to the prevention of teratogenicity, since the principal time of organogenesis is during the first ten weeks. In practice it is unusual for pregnant women to have infections detected, let alone treated, before the fifteenth week of pregnancy. Therefore, in order to make a logical approach to prevention of fetal abnormalities due to chemotherapy it would be necessary to ban any antimicrobial drug under suspicion to all women liable to become pregnant, in order to prevent administration in early pregnancy.

It has already been inferred that translation of toxicity data from the animal to the human situation is dangerous. For instance, patients suffering from disseminated lupus erythematosus treated with azathioprine (Imuran, B.W. & Co.) have, until recently, been advised not to become pregnant since the score of fetal abnormalities in rats given azathioprine was very high. However, recently a few patients receiving azathioprine for the treatment of disseminated lupus erythematosus have become pregnant and, in spite of therapy with azathioprine throughout pregnancy, have delivered normal infants.[27]

Antibiotics in Renal Failure

Antibiotics can be extremely dangerous in renal failure if they are dependent on the renal route of excretion. Some antimicrobials excreted by this route can, however, be administered with only minor modification in dosage,[28,29] whereas others need both major modification of dosage and continuous monitoring of the blood level.[30]

Nitrofurantoin should never be given in renal failure because of the high risk of toxicity and amphotericin B should be avoided

---

TABLE IX

A General Guide to Modification of Antibiotic Dosage in the Presence of Impaired Renal Function

	Modification in dose
Penicillins Cephalosporins Erythromycin Chloramphenicol Fusidic acid	Minor
Tetracyclines Aminoglycosides Polymyxin Colistin Cycloserine	Major
Amphotericin B Nitrofurantoin	Avoid

when an alternative is available. A quantitative guide to the modification of dose required for a variety of antibiotics that may be used in renal failure is summarized in Table IX.

Conclusions

Antibiotics are, on the whole, extremely safe compounds, and with correct use and modification of dosage it is possible to use these substances without danger to the patient. Most complications would be avoided if a history were taken from the patient and precipitating causes of trouble, such as impairment of renal function, anticipated. Unfortunately, one of the more serious reasons for adverse reaction to antibiotics is their widespread use in seriously ill patients when there is no proper indication. If the use of antibiotics were discontinued for conditions such as virus respiratory infections and glandular fever, where they have no therapeutic value, a number of needless adverse reactions would be avoided.

REFERENCES

1. Odell GB: The dissociation of bilirubin from albumin and its clinical implications. J Pediat 55:269-279, 1959.
2. Dunn PM: The possible relationship between maternal administration of sulfamethoxypyridiazine and hyperbilirubinaemia in the newborn. J Obstet Gynaec Brit Cwlth 71:128-131, 1964.
3. Adamson K Jr and Joelsson J: The effects of pharmacological agents upon the fetus and newborn. Amer J Obstet Gynec 96:437-460, 1966.
4. Dujovne CA, Chan CH and Zimmerman HJ: Sulfonamide hepatic injury. Review of the literature and report of a case due to sulfamethoxazole. NEJM 277:758-785, 1967.
5. Harris MJ, Wise G and Beveridge J; The Stevens-Johnson syndrome and long-acting sulphonamides. Aust Paed J 2:103-109, 1966.
6. Beveridge J: Personal Communication.
7. Wereide K:. The Stevens-Johnson syndrome in Norway with particular reference to its relation to sulfhonamides. Vth Int Congr Chemotherapy, Ed Spitzy KH, Haschak H, Verlag der Weiner Medizinischen Akademie Vol IV, 421-426, 1967.
8. Bianchine JR, Macaraeg PVJ, Lasagna L, et al: Drugs as etiologic factors in the Stevens-Johnson syndrome. Am J Med 44:390-405, 1968.
9. Gruneberg RN and Brumfitt W: Single-dose treatment of acute urinary tract infection: a controlled trial. Brit Med J 3:649-651, 1967.
10. Shapiro S, Slone D, Siskind V, et al: Drug rash with ampicillin and other penicillins. Lancet 2:969-972, 1969.
11. Ley AB, Harris JP, Brinkley M, et al: Circulating antibody directed against penicillin. Science 127:1118-1119, 1958.
12. Shelley WB: Indirect basophile degranulation test for allergy to penicillin and other drugs. J Amer Med Ass 184:171-178, 1963.
13. Halpern B and Amache N: Diagnosis of drug allergy in vitro with the lymphocyte transformation test. J Allergy 40:168-181, 1967.
14. Katz HI, Gill KA, Baxter DL. et al: Indirect basophile degranulation test in penicillin allergy. J Amer Med Ass 18:351-354, 1964.
15. DeWeck AL and Eisen HN: Some immunochemical properties of penicillenic acid. An antigenic determinant derived from penicillin. J Exp Med 112:1227-1247, 1960.
16. Resnick SS and Shelley WB: Penicillcyl-polylysine skin test: anaphylaxis in absence of penicillin sensitivity. J Amer Med Ass 196:750. 1966.
17. Pullen H, Wright N and Murdock JMcC: Hypersensitivity reactions to antibacterial drugs in infectious mononucleosis. Lancet 2:1177-1178, 1967.
18. Geddes AM: Personal communication.
19. Brown JJ, Gleadle RI, Lawson DH, et al: Renin and acute renal failure: studies in man. Brit Med J 1:253-258, 1970.
20. Foord R: Personal communication.
21. Davies R: Personal communication.
22. Ackroyd JF: Personal communication.
23. Robinson MM: Antibiotics increase the incidence of hepatitis. J Amer Med Ass 178:89, 1961.
24. Kohlstaedt KG: Propionyl erythromycin ester lauryl sulfate and jaundice. J Amer Med Ass 178:89-90, 1961.
25. Udall V: Toxicology of sulfonamide-trimethoprim combination. Postgrad Med J 45. suppl:42-45, 1969.
26. Williams JD, Brumfitt W, Condie AP, et al: The treatment of bacteriuria in pregnant women with sulphamethoxazole and trimethoprim. Postgrad Med J 45, suppl:71-75, 1969.
27. Peart WS: Personal communication.
28. Williams DMJ, Winpenny J and Asscher AW: Renal clearance of sodium sulfadimidine in normal and uraemic subjects. Lancet 2:1058-1060, 1968.
29. Sharpstone P: The renal handling of trimethoprim and sulfamethoxazole in man. Postgrad Med J 45, suppl:38-42, 1969.
30. Kunin CM: A guide to use of antibiotics in patients with renal disease. Ann Intern Med 67:151-158, 1967.

INFECTIONS DUE TO NON-SPOREFORMING ANAEROBIC BACTERIA

• Non-sporeforming anaerobic bacteria undoubtedly cause many infections but the diagnosis is often missed because they are not suspected and because culture techniques are not adequate.

SYDNEY M. FINEGOLD, M.D.

Infections with non-sporulating anaerobes are found relatively often when clinicians and bacteriologists are aware of their importance and proper bacteriologic techniques are used. Thus Lodeṇkämper and Stienen[1] diagnosed 690 anaerobic infections during an eight-year period. Of these, 239 yielded gram-negative anaerobic bacilli in pure culture. Stokes[2] found anaerobes in over 10% of 4,737 positive cultures from all types of clinical material. In this series, purulent exudate from abdominal and genital infections yielded anaerobes in essentially one-third of the specimens. Gram-negative non-sporeforming anaerobic bacilli and anaerobic cocci were present in equal numbers and together accounted for almost 90% of the anaerobes isolated. Only one in 15 anaerobic isolates was a *Clostridium*.

The present report will not consider gram-positive non-sporulating anaerobes and their role in infectious processes since these organisms are found much less commonly than other non-sporulating anaerobes, since their classification is very much uncertain at present, and since good information on the most commonly encountered organisms of this group *(Actinomyces)* and related infections is readily available.

Infections Due to Gram-negative Anaerobic

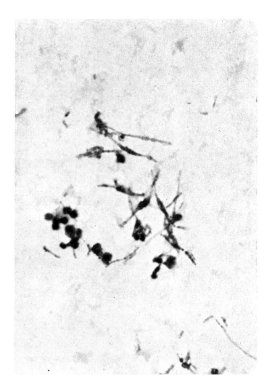

Figure 1

Microscopic morphology Sphaerophorus. Note filaments with swellings along course, large round bodies, and irregularity of staining.*
*From Medical Times 96:174, 1968.

Dr. Finegold is Chief, Infectious Disease Section, Wadsworth Veterans Administration Hospital, Los Angeles, California.

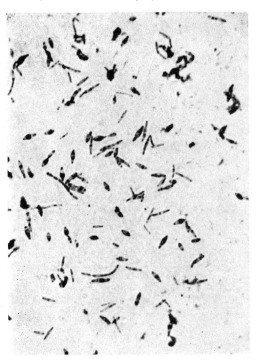

Figure 2

Microscopic morphology B. fragilis. Note pleomorphism and irregular staining.*

*From The Anaerobic Bacteria, proceedings of an International Workshop held at the University of Montreal, 1968. Edited by V. Fredette.

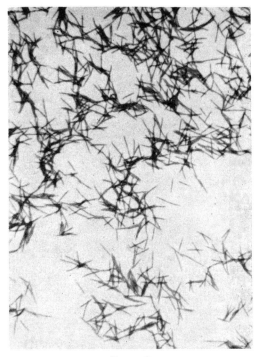

Figure 3

Microscopic morphology F. fusiforme. Note the long, thin bacilli with tapered ends.*

*From The Anaerobic Bacteria, proceedings of an International Workshop held at the University of Montreal, 1968. Edited by V. Fredette.

Bacilli. — The organisms in this group are presently classified in three major genera: *Bacteroides, Sphaerophorus,* and *Fusobacterium.* Several species are encountered frequently — *B. fragilis, B. melaninogenicus (B. nigrescens), B. oralis, S. necrophorus (F. necrophorus, B. funduliformis), S. mortiferus, S. varius* and *F. fusiforme. B. fragilis* is isolated much more often than the others, perhaps partly related to the fact that it is less fastidious. Although *B. oralis* is encountered in clinical material occasionally, together with other organisms, its role in infection is uncertain.

These organisms commonly display unique microscopic or colonial morphology; this may allow the clinician and bacteriologist to suspect their presence when examining gram stains of exudates or cultures. Carbol fuchsin is the counterstain of choice for the gram stain when these organisms may be present; even with it, however, this group characteristically stains lightly. Irregularity of staining (light and dark areas scattered randomly) is also characteristic. Members of the genus *Sphaerophorus* are usually the most pleomorphic of the group, often showing filamentous forms, swellings along the filaments, and detached large round bodies (Figure 1). *B. fragilis* (Figure 2) and *B. oralis* are usually less pleomorphic and less distinctive. *F. fusiforme* (Figure 3) usually stains evenly and is not pleomorphic, but is very distinctive in that it occurs as thin, long bacilli with tapered ends; often organisms appear in pairs. *B. melaninogenicus* may be bacillary and pleomorphic but most often occurs as regularly staining coccobacilli (Figure 4); its most distinctive feature

18

Number of Cases	Type of Infection
12	Bacteremia
1	Subacute bacterial endocarditis
2	Urinary tract infection
14	Peritonitis
29	Intra-abdominal abscess
27	Other abscesses (including lung, brain, liver, breast, ovarian, subcutaneous)
26	Wound infection (chiefly following bowel surgery)
11	Thoracic empyema
19	Miscellaneous infections (including meningitis, mastoiditis, pylephlebitis, pneumonia, osteomyelitis and endometritis)
141	

TABLE 1

CLINICAL EXPERIENCE WITH GRAM-NEGATIVE ANAEROBIC BACILLI

Modified from Finegold SM and Hewitt WL: *Proc VIII International Congress for Microbiology*, Montreal, E 35.2, 1962.

is the brown-black colonial pigment developing on blood-containing media (Figure 5).

The gram-negative abnaeroic bacilli form a prominent part of the normal endogenous

TABLE 2

ANAEROBIC COCCAL INFECTIONS

	No. CASES
Subacute bacterial endocarditis	10
Bacteremia	2
Brain abscess	5
Liver abscess	3
Pneumonia, lung abscess, empyema	12
Intra-abdominal abscess	6
Peritonitis	2
Pelvic abscess, Bartholin abscess, septic abortion	3
Perirectal abscess, infected pilonidal cyst	4
Wound infection (following bowel surgery, nephrostomy, etc.)	7
Soft tissue infections (some with gas in tissues)	16
Osteomyelitis	6
Suppurative myositis	1
Maxillary sinusitis	1
Infected human bite	1
	79

Modified from Finegold, Miller, and Sutter. *Bacteriol Proc* 94, 1968.

flora of man. They are present on essentially all mucous membrane surfaces of the body — the mouth, upper respiratory tract, gastrointestinal tract and the genital tract. In the colon, these organisms (particularly *B. fragilis*) are the predominant element of the flora, outnumbering *E. coli* 1000 to one.[3] They play a role in certain pathophysiologic processes such as the blind loop syndrome.[4]

These organisms also cause a variety of infections of virtually all types, mostly in proximity to the mucosal surfaces where they exist normally. Table 1 summarizes our clinical experiences with infections involving gram-negative anaerobic bacilli.[5] These organisms were isolated in pure culture in one-third of the cases, with *B. fragilis* the most common isolate. In mixed infections, a variety of other anaerobes and aerobes are encountered. X-rays from three of the patients in our series are shown in Figure 6, 7 and 8.

A number of these infections were very difficult to manage and led to prolonged hospitalization and disability and, at times, to extensive tissue destruction and death. Abscess formation was common, and septic thrombophlebitis was encountered occasionally. A number of the infections, particularly among those related to the gastrointestinal tract,

19

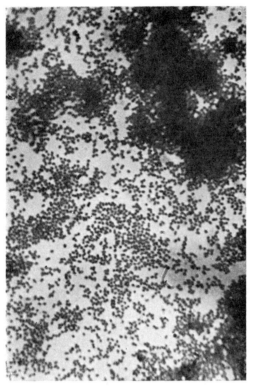

Figure 4

Microscopic, morphology B. melaninogenicus. Organisms are coccobacilli.*

*Reproduced from Gradwohl's Clinical Laboratory Methods and Diagnosis, 7th Edition, C.V. Mosby Co., St. Louis, Mo.

were associated with malignancy. Some followed systemic or topical use of kanamycin or neomycin, agents to which this group (and anaerobes generally) are quite resistant.

The patient with subacute bacterial endocarditis was a particular problem. The infecting organism was *B. fragilis*, and it was not possible to find an antibiotic or combination of antibiotics with clinically significant bactericidal activity against it. Remissions were obtained repeatedly, usually with a combination of tetracycline and erythromycin, but despite prolonged courses of therapy (some exceeding three months) the patient would always relapse clinically and bacteriologically soon after therapy was discontinued. The patient ultimately died after over two years of intermittent treatment.

Infections Due to Anaerobic Cocci

Present classification systems for these organisms are not entirely satisfactory. However, for clinical purposes, it is usually adequate to note whether they are cocci (in pairs or masses) or streptococci, whether they are obligately anaerobic or microaerophilic, what type of hemolysis is produced (if any), and whether they are gram-positive or gram-negative. Anaerobic cocci are also widely distributed as normal flora in humans; compared to the gram-negative anaerobic bacilli, the cocci are more prevalent in the genital and

TABLE 3

SUSCEPTIBILITY OF NON-SPORULATING ANAEROBES TO CLINICALLY USEFUL ANTIBIOTICS

	Anaerobic Cocci	Bacteroides fragilis	Sphaerophorus	Other Bacteroides and Fusobacterium
Penicillin G	+ + + +*	+	+ + +*	+ + + +
Tetracycline	+ +	+ + + +	+ + +	+ + +
Chloramphenicol	+ + +	+ + +	+ + +	+ + +
Lincomycin	+ + +	+ to + +	+ + +**	+ + +
Erythromycin	+ + +	+ +	+	+ to + +
Vancomycin	+ + +	+	+	+

* + + + + Drug of choice   + Poor or inconsistent activity
+ + + Good activity   + + Moderate activity
** Few strains resistant

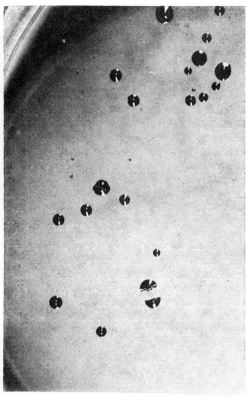

Figure 5

Colony morphology B. melaninogenicus. Note black pigment.*
*From Medical Times 96:174, 1968.

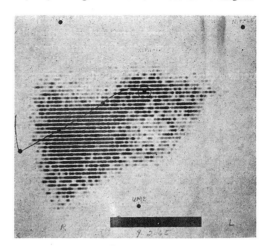

Figure 6-A

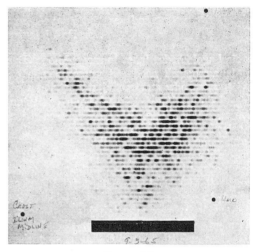

Figure 6-B

A-P and lateral Au[198] liver scan from patient with microaerophilic streptococcal liver abscess, showing a large space-occupying lesion in the upper right lobe.*
*From Annals of Surgery 165:362, 1967.

upper respiratory tracts and relatively scarce in the gastrointestinal tract.

The microscopic morphology of anaerobic cocci is not very unique; however, they are often tiny or distinctly smaller than aerobic (facultative) forms.

In general, the anaerobic cocci produce infections similar to those produced by the gram-negative anaerobic bacilli with differences related to the above-mentioned differences in distribution in the body. Two other major differences in types of infection encountered are a much greater incidence of subacute bacterial endocarditis (10% of our cases of subacute endocarditis over a ten-year period were due to anaerobic cocci) and the capability of anaerobic cocci to produce sup-

purative myositis. Our clinical experience with these organisms[6] is given in Table 2. As with the gram-negative anaerobic bacilli, anaerobic cocci were isolated in pure culture from one-third of the infections in which they were involved. Figure 6A, B shows liver scans from a patient with liver abscess, and Figure 7 shows the gram stain of the pus obtained from

21

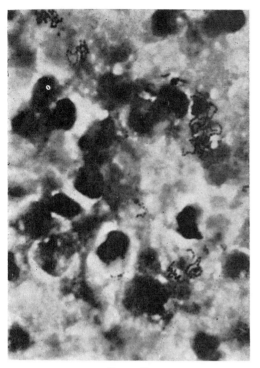

Figure 7

Gram stain of pus from the liver abscess shown in Figure 9. Note the chains of small cocci. (Magnification x 1000)

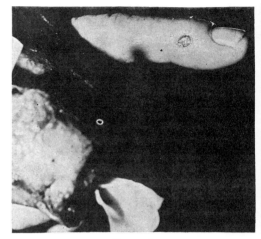

Figure 8

Mixed infection of finger due to anaerobic streptococcus and S. aureus. Precipitating event unknown. Partial amputation, through and through incision and drainage, and chemotherapy led to cure.

this abscess at surgery; microaerophilic streptococci were isolated in pure culture. Figure 8 shows extensive edema and tissue destruction in a finger involved in a mixed infection with anaerobic streptococci and *S. aureus.*

Diagnosis of Anaerobic Infections

The frequency of diagnosis of these infections varies directly with the knowledge and interest of clinicians and bacteriologists. The use of anaerobic jars or even better anaerobic systems is imperative. Five to 10% carbon dioxide must be provided in the atmosphere. Many smaller laboratories use fluid thioglycollate medium as the only procedure for isolation of anaerobes; this is entirely inadequate. The commercial blood culture bottles presently recommended for anaerobic culture are unsatisfactory. Screw-capped blood culture bottles (without a rubber diaphragm) should be incubated, with the caps loosened, in an anaerobic jar.

The most important clinical clue to the possible presence of anaerobes in infection is foul-smelling discharge; this essentially always means anaerobes are involved. Other tip-offs include location of infection near a mucosal surface, necrotic tissue or gangrene, gas in tissues or discharges, infection associated with malignancy or other process producing tissue destruction, infection related to the systemic or topical use of kanamycin or related agents, septic thrombophlebitis, infection following bites, subacute bacterial endocarditis with negative blood cultures, gram stain of discharge showing characteristic organisms, failure of the laboratory to recover on routine culture organisms seen on direct smear, or total absence of growth from purulent exudate. The importance of the gram stain cannot be overemphasized; it alerts one to the possibility of anaerobic infection, it serves as a check on culture technique, and it provides a tentative bacteriologic diagnosis two to

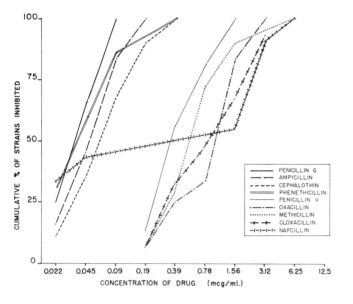

Figure 9

Activity of penicillin-like drugs vs.
B. melaninogenicus.*

*From Medical Times 96:174, 1968.

three days or more before even preliminary cultural results are available.

There are two problems to be kept in mind with regard to collection of specimens from patients with possible anaerobic infection. Care must be taken to avoid "contamination" with normal anaerobic flora. In the case of pulmonary infections, the normal mouth and pharyngeal flora may best be bypassed by means of transtracheal puncture, and with urinary tract infections (anaerobes are not often involved in these), percutaneous bladder puncture bypasses the normal urethral flora.[7] Other types of infections may present a challenge for means to avoid normal flora. The other problem concerns maintaining anaerobiosis from the time a specimen is obtained until it is cultured anaerobically, so that the more fastidious anaerobes will not die off. Displacing all of the air in a screw-capped Wasserman tube with the specimen works well. With smaller specimens, place in tube with atmosphere of oxygen-free gas by means of syringe and needle.[8]

Therapeutic Considerations

Drainage of collections of pus and excision of necrotic tissue are extremely important as-
pects of therapy. Hydrogen peroxide may be useful as a local measure, and hyperbaric oxygen may play a role in unusual infections involving non-sporulating anaerobes.

The susceptibility of various non-sporeforming anaerobes to the most useful antibiotics is noted in Table 3. Penicillin G is the most active of these drugs and exhibits the best bactericidal activity; it is the drug of choice for all anaerobic infections except those due to *B. fragilis* and to strains of *Sphaerophorus* resistant to it. Other penicillins and the cephalosporins are usually less active than penicillin G and sometimes have no clinically useful activity. This is illustrated, for *B. melaninogenicus*, in Figure 9. The degree of activity of various penicillins and cephalosporins varies with the type of organism, but ampicillin and cephaloridine generally approach penicillin G in activity.

Summary

Infections due to non-sporulating anaerobes are at least ten times as common as those due to *clostridia* and undoubtedly represent the most frequently undiagnosed or misdiagnosed of the bacterial infections. These anaerobes (chiefly gram-negative bacilli and gram-positive cocci) may cause virtually any type of infection in any area of the body. Major clues suggesting the possibility of anaerobic infection include foul-smelling discharge, gas in tissues, tissue necrosis, absence of growth in routine culture despite presence of organisms on direct smear, and the unique morphology of certain of these organisms on gram stain. Diagnostic difficulties relate to unawareness of these anaerobes and failure to maintain anaerobiosis or to exclude normal flora when obtaining specimens. Drainage of abscesses and excision of necrotic tissue are important therapeutic considerations. Antibiotics most useful are tetracycline, chloramphenicol, penicillin G and lincomycin.

REFERENCES

1. Lodenkamper H and Stienen G: Importance and therapy of anaerobic infections. Antibiotic Med 1:653-660, 1955.
2. Stokes EJ: Anaerobes in routine diagnostic cultures. Lancet 1:668-670, 1958.
3. Finegold SM and Miller LG: Normal fecal flora of adult humans. Bacteriol Proc 93, 1968
4. Polter DE, Boyle JD, Miller LG, et al: Anaerobic bacteria as cause of the blind loop syndrome: A case with observations on response to antibacterial agents. Gastroenterology 54:1148-1154, 1968.
5. Finegold SM and Hewitt WL: Laboratory and clinical features of infections due to gram-negative, non-sporeforming anaerobic bacilli. Proc VIII Intern Congress for Microbiology, Montreal, E35.2, 1962.
6. Finegold, SM, Miller AB and Sutter VL: Anaerobic cocci in human infection. Bacteriol Proc 94, 1968.
7. Finegold SM, Miller LG. Merrill SL, et al. The significance of anaerobic and capnophilic bacteria isolated from the urinary tract, Kass EH ed. Progress in Pyelonephritis, Philadelphia, FA Davis 159-178, 1965
8. Attebery HR and Finegold SM: Combined screwcap and rubber-stopper closure for hungate tubes (prereduced, anaerobically sterilized roll tubes and liquid media). Applied Microbiol 18:558-561, 1969.

TULAREMIA IN HAMSTER HUNTERS

• Tularemia is one of the most common examples of zoonosis presenting in medical practice today. Accurate diagnosis is enhanced if the clinician is aware of the presence of the disease in his locale.

JOSEPH SZEKELYFOLDI, M.D.

The first cases of tularemia in central Europe occurred in Marchfeld in 1936-1937. In neighboring western Hungary, the first infection was not seen until 1951. Since then cases have been seen regularly, and the source has been wild rabbits.

In our area of Hungary, which is 300 miles from the area of recurring infections, the first cases were seen in 1966 when eighteen cases were diagnosed. In each case, the source of the infection was hamsters.

Hamsters are hunted for their precious skin, especially in spring and autumn when the fur is heaviest. Humans handling the hamsters may be infected in various ways. The hunter who removes the hamster from the trap may be bitten and thus infected. Others are scratched by the teeth in the process of skinning the animal, as the skin is removed around the head. Individuals may also be infected while handling the skin as it is dried. In addition, contact with the ectoparasites of the rodent and any food or water contaminated by the animal, for instance, field products such as sugar beets, may be the source of the organisms. One epidemic in 1966 was even traced to breathing contaminated air in a sugar factory where the beets were being processed.

We investigated this epidemic to determine how the infection came to our area, if there were asymptomatic cases and how the infection might be prevented.

All of our patients were hamster hunters. The disease first occurred in the first and fourth quarters of 1966. The disease was localized in four villages beside the Berettyo River. Only one of the eighteen cases was a woman, and all patients were over twenty years old.

The affected hand was usually the left, and the area of the wound was painful. There was lymphangitis up to the axilla, which also contained swollen, painful lymph nodes. Diagnosis was confirmed by both a serum agglutination test and a positive skin test. The patients were all treated with tetracycline and streptomycin. All symptoms quickly disappeared except for the swollen lymph nodes, which slowly decreased in size.

Since all of the cases were in hamster hunters, we considered why the hamsters in our area were suddenly infected. There was no importing of rabbits from the western areas, considered endemic. Other known reservoirs such as mice, rats, hares and limmings did not appear to be the source. It seems probable that the infected hamsters came to us from bordering Rumanian areas along the Berettyo, since our epidemic was confined to the river area. Tularemia has been found in hamster hunters in Rumania, with an epidemic reported in 1955 by Mr. Condrea.

To confirm that the infection was confined to the river area and to determine how widespread the infection was among our hamster hunters, we did the tularin skin test. This test has been reported by Jirovec to be positive in individuals who have had tularemia for as long as 15-17 years after the infection.

We tested 324 handlers of hamsters in twenty villages in the area. The skin test was read 48 hours after application of the

Dr. Szekelyfoldi is from Nyiregyhara Megyei korhaz, Hungary.

tularin. Twenty individuals, 6.1%, gave a positive reaction. Three of these had had the cutaneous, glandular infection in 1965 and three others in 1966. At the time of testing, a residue of clinical symptoms could be found, but none were treated. Nine others reported no history of symptoms, and it is supposed that the infection was subclinical.

An investigation by Ljung[1] revealed that 11% of a population not selected for an epidemic had positive tularin skin tests and that 90% of those known to be infected gave a positive test. Because of our lower incidence, 6.1%, we concluded that we have no group infected in previous years and that the infection was introduced to our area shortly before the first infections were seen in 1965.

The association of the infection with hamsters suggests the measures needed to prevent further infections. The hunters have been warned that a bite or scratch during skinning may lead to disease. It has been suggested that a defending thimble be used while handling or skinning the animals. They have also been told to see a doctor at once if they notice swollen lymph nodes and a high fever.

The doctors have been alerted to think of tularemia when they see swollen lymph nodes and to confirm diagnosis by the blood test and skin test.

The most important preventive measure would be the vaccination of the hamster catchers. The scarification tularemia vaccination immunizes for five years. Permission for catching hamsters could be denied until vaccination has been obtained.

REFERENCE
1. Ljung O: Intraermal and agglutination tests in tularemia; with particular regard to the demonstration of past infection. Acta Med Scand 161(1):149-154, 1958.

CARBENICILLIN IN PULMONARY INFECTION COMPLICATING CYSTIC FIBROSIS

• Carbenicillin appears to be an effective agent for the treatment of pseudomonas infections in patients with cystic fibrosis.

Eva Africa, M.D.
Herman Rosenblum, M.D.

The predominant organism recovered from throat and sputum cultures of patients with cystic fibrosis is currently a *Pseudomonas aeruginosa*. The sputum and throat cultures of the patients attending Cystic Fibrosis Clinic of the Wilmington Medical Center are currently being studied to evaluate the bacterial flora as an aid in the selection of the appropriate antibiotic.* The antibiotic carbenicillin is currently being evaluated as an agent in the therapy of *Pseudomonas aeruginosa* infections and specifically in cystic fibrosis patients.

We should like to present the case summaries of these four patients with cystic fibrosis who were admitted in respiratory distress to the Department of Pediatrics of the Wilmington Medical Center. These patients were all treated with carbenicillin, either alone or in combination with cephalothin. The clinical response was good in all four patients with temporary alleviation of symptoms and in one patient marked improvement of the chest x-ray.

A fifteen-year-old white boy, had been diagnosed as having cystic fibrosis at the age of three years. He was first admitted to the Wilmington Medical Center on June 27, 1969, because of fatigue of two months' duration,

cough and fever. Prior to admission his antibiotic therapy consisted of oxacillin, 500 mg, and tetracycline, 250 mg three times a day, respectively. One week prior to admission his temperature ranged from 100-102°.

On admission he appeared chronically and acutely ill and dyspneic. Examination of his lungs revealed rales bilaterally. There was 4+ clubbing of the fingers. A sputum culture was taken prior to antibiotic therapy and revealed a marked increase in *Pseudomonas aeruginosa* which was sensitive to carbenicillin. A chest x-ray revealed several bilateral changes with fibrosis and areas of infiltration. He was treated with intravenous carbenicillin, 500 mg/kg/day in twelve divided doses for fourteen days. His clinical response was excellent, he became and remained afebrile throughout his hospitalization. Dyspnea subsided, cough became minimal and rales were not heard after clinical improvement became evident. There was marked improvement in the chest x-ray.

About eight and one-half months later he was readmitted because of sharp chest pain on respiration and tachypnea of a few days' duration. On physical examination he appeared chronically and acutely ill, dyspneic and tachypneic. He was coughing incessantly and there were disseminated rales in his chest. Respiratory rate was 40 per minute. His sputum culture showed a *Pseudomonas aeruginosa* which was sensitive to carbenicil-

Dr. Africa is Resident in Pediatrics and Dr. Rosenblum is Coordinator of Education and Clinical Services, Department of Pediatrics, Wilmington Medical Center, Wilmington, Delaware.

* Supported by a grant from the National Cystic Fibrosis Research Foundation.

lin. He again received a fourteen-day course of I. V. carbenicillin, 500 mg/kg/day in twelve divided doses. Response to therapy was again excellent both clinically and in improvement of his x-ray.

A three and one-half year old white girl was diagnosed as having cystic fibrosis at the age of six months. She was admitted to the Delaware Division for the first time on November 13, 1968, because of tachypnea, cough and wheezing of one day's duration. On physical examination she appeared acutely ill, coughing continuously and tachypneic. Examination of the lungs revealed expiratory wheezes and rales at both lung bases. A throat culture revealed a *Pseudomonas aeruginosa* sensitive to carbenicillin and a *Staphylococcus aureus* resistant to penicillin. Chest x-ray revealed extensive diffuse infiltrates throughout both lung fields. Treatment consisted of carbenicillin, 300 mg/kg/BW/day for a total of eight and one-half days. A throat culture taken after completion of therapy revealed a normal flora. Her appetite improved once her cough had subsided, and she gained one pound of body weight during her hospital stay. Her clinical response was considered good.

A nine-month-old white boy, was diagnosed as a case of cystic fibrosis at the age of two months. On July 8, 1968, he was admitted for the second time to the Delaware Division because of failure to thrive and tachypnea. He was receiving Prostaphlin (Bristol) as an outpatient. About one month prior to admission he developed a cough and was failing to gain weight. On admission he looked chronically ill, was tachypneic with a respiratory rate of 60 per minute. Auscultation of the lungs revealed no rales, but breath sounds were increased in intensity. Chest x-ray revealed hyperaeration. Throat culture revealed normal flora. Despite the normal flora in the throat culture it was decided to treat him with carbenicillin, 200 mg/kg/day. After 10 days of I. V. carbenicillin, he was discharged markedly improved, without tachypnea and having gained one pound of body weight.

Our fourth case is that of an eight-month-old white boy who was admitted in November of 1969 for failure to thrive, vomiting and tachypnea. This infant had had feeding problems since birth for which multiple changes in formula had been made. At six months of age a sweat chloride was obtained which revealed a value of 31 mEq/L. He was presumed to have a cow's milk allergy. On admission he appeared chronically and acutely ill, tachypneic, grunting with respiration rate of 36 per minute and a weight of 12 pounds, 6 ounces. Examination of the chest revealed diffuse rales. He developed rectal prolapse which prompted re-evaluation of the sweat chlorides which on two occasions gave values of 91 mEq/L and 121 mEq/L. On December 3, 1969, a throat culture revealed 50% *Pseudomonas aeruginosa* sensitive to carbenicillin, gentamicin and tetracycline and 20% *Klebsiella aerogenes* resistant to carbenicillin but sensitive to cephalothin. With this sensitivity study, it was decided to treat him with a 14-day course of I. V. carbenicillin, 300 mg/kg/day and cephalothin. Response to therapy was excellent.

In summary, the case histories of four patients with cystic fibrosis and pulmonary complications are presented. The results of carbenicillin therapy are encouraging for at least temporary improvement of the symptoms.

KIDNEY TUBERCULOSIS

• Effective antimicrobial therapy has lowered the incidence of renal tuberculosis and obviated the need for a surgical approach to the problem. A high index of suspicion is still necessary for diagnosis.

JOHN K. LATTIMER, M.D., Sc.D.

Renal tuberculosis can still destroy the kidneys in three or four years, if unrecognized, and untreated. We have had cases where it destroyed them rapidly and insidiously, causing very few symptoms.

While the incidence of renal tuberculosis in native Americans is at least showing signs of a decline, we have so many patients arriving in our port cities, and the giant airplane is bringing in so many visitors, that we are bound to have a continuing tuberculosis problem.

Fortunately, this serious complication of tuberculosis can now almost always be controlled with nonoperative therapy. Persistent specific chemotherapy, combined with conscientious monitoring by cystoscopic, x-ray and laboratory examinations, has gradually permitted medicines to supplant the knife, in the years since 1946. Eighteen years of faithful follow-up observations on several hundred cases of this relatively rare disease by the Research Unit for Genitourinary Tuberculosis of the Kingsbridge Veterans Administration Hospital and the Columbia University Department of Urology appear to justify this position. For example, in one group of 333 patients in whom the effects of chemotherapy alone could be well evaluated, it was possible eventually to arrest every case, regardless of the extent or activity of the disease, by the persistent reapplication of new combinations of drugs to the patients who relapsed. Fifteen per cent of the patients required two, 5% three, and 1% four regimens of treatment.[1]

Careful attention to the principle of multiple-drug (three drugs) administration and long-term (two years) duration of each regimen was necessary to achieve this result. At the two hospitals involved, the Presbyterian Hospital and the Kingsbridge Veterans Administration Hospital in New York City, it has not been necessary to do any nephrectomies because of tuberculosis for the past seven years. The only two tuberculous kidneys that were removed within this period at either hospital were in children, of whom one had a tuberculous mass that could not be differentiated with certainty from a Wilms' tumor, and the other the thin-walled shell of a previously tuberculous kidney, which was removed in an effort to stimulate more rapid compensatory hypertrophy on the contralateral side. In neither case was progression of the tuberculosis the reason for the nephrectomy. It is acknowledged that intractable pain or secondary infection behind a tuberculous ureteral stricture might force a nephrectomy to be done, but no such cases have been encountered in seven years.

One group of 22 large, nonfunctioning tuberculous kidneys was left in place when the urine had become negative after chemotherapy, and neither relapses nor complications such as hypertension have yet developed in this group, which has now been observed for an average of seven years.[2] It should be noted that after surveying a similar group of patients treated in England, one observer still suggested that traditional excisional therapy should be utilized for large lesions, even though his most modern chemotherapy had brought about superb (total) conversions of

Dr. Lattimer is Professor and Chairman, Department of Urology, Columbia, College of Physicians and Surgeons, and Director, Squier Urological Clinic.

the urine in 200 cases whereas nephrectomy had converted only one out of six.[3]

Scattered reports of small series of cases from other points in the world suggest that multiple-drug, long-term chemotherapy is indeed effective but that occasional patients may require either extraordinary persistence and reapplication of chemotherapy or ultimate excision. There appears to be some belief that excision after chemotherapy might shorten the period of treatment or morbidity, but there is no proof of this, and the necessity for prolonged and conscientious follow-up examinations still would not be avoided. In my opinion the follow-up examinations would be necessary even if excision was added.

Effective Orally Administered Medications

The advent of such effective antituberculosis agents as isoniazid, sodium para-aminosalicylic acid (PAS), ethambutol, ethionamide and cycloserine has made it possible to put aside injectable drugs such as streptomycin, dihydrostreptomycin, viomycin and kanamycin, except for the retreatment of refractory cases. Regimens consisting of isoniazid, 100 mg three times daily, and sodium PAS, 5 gm three times daily, given continuously over a two-year period, have brought about seven-year conversion rates of the order of 81% on the first attempt. It should be noted that any long-term isoniazid regimen should be accompanied by pyridoxine, 50 mg twice daily, as a preventive against possible neuritis. It has been the custom of this research unit to combine six months of semiambulatory bed rest with the beginning of the two-year treatment, but this has not proved to be an essential measure.[4]

Similar groups given triple-drug treatment, over a two-year period, have consistently yielded slightly higher percentages of conversions, two, five and eight years after the beginning of treatment, than the comparable groups of patients treated with only two drugs.[5] The advantage of the triple-drug groups over the two-drug groups has been statistically significant only at about the 5% level, however. It has been suggested that this apparent slight superiority might represent the fact that some patients tend to skip doses of a drug with annoying side effects, such as sodium PAS, whereas they might continue to take less toxic drugs such as isoniazid or cycloserine without interruption (there is a tradition to the effect that outside every sanatorium window there is a patch where the grass will not grow because of the PAS pills that were thrown out by the more sophisticated patients). The fact that a two-drug regimen would suffer severely in efficacy if the PAS were omitted, whereas a triple-drug regimen would suffer a great deal less from this same omission, might account for the statistical difference in the two groups of patients. Further evidence for the efficacy of the two-drug treatment, when taken faithfully, appears when the comparisons of the two-drug and triple-drug regimens are confined only to the cases showing a high output of tubercle bacilli in the urine. In this comparison the two become approximately equal in efficacy.

Responsiveness of renal tuberculous lesions to chemotherapy has been demonstrated to be much poorer in patients who are putting out large numbers of tubercle bacilli in the urine, so that more than one of their twenty-four-hour concentrates is positive. Patients who have produced only an isolated positive urine culture are much more likely to respond to chemotherapy according to the work of Segawa and Reilly.[1] This bacteriologic activity is even more important than the magnitude and extent of the lesions in the kidney, in deciding prognosis. Although massive cavitary lesions may be more difficult to arrest than minimal lesions (in which no cavity can be seen), the extent of destruction proved less important than the bacteriologic activity, in predicting response to treatment.

Conscientious ureteral calibration is necessary if ureteral strictures are to be avoided. Although intravenous pyelography every six months during the first five years of treatment will indicate widening of the ureter as an evidence of stricture formation, the passage of a No. 6 Fr. ureteral catheter up and down the ureters every six months is both diagnostic and therapeutic at the same time and at an earlier stage. Tuberculous contractures of the bladder were seen in a surprising 7% of these patients, and whereas some responded to chemotherapy, combined with a stretching of the bladder by hydraulic dilatation, others required enlargement of the bladder by an addition of a patch of intestinal wall. This could only be done when the ureterovesical valve had not been destroyed, so that there was no reflux to the kidneys.

It was apparent that the majority of relapses would occur within two years after the chemotherapeutic treatment and that almost all the additional relapses would occur before five years of follow-up study, and no additional relapses have ocurred after eight years of diligent follow-up observation in the eighteen years of experience of this research unit.

It was of interest that the children of these patients, who were exposed only to the tuberculous urine of their parents, had positive skin tests in 22%, as compared with traditional control-group rates of 4% to 10%.[6] Thus, the necessity for placing patients suspected of having active urinary tuberculosis on precautions is emphasized. This practice is not widely followed at the present time.

Instrument Sterilization

Cold sterilization of cystoscopes, as traditionally done, is woefully inadequate, according to the findings of this group. Oxycyanide of mercury, for example, either in 1:1000 or even 1:100 concentrations, quarternary ammonium compounds (widely sold for sterilizing cystoscopes), and newer iodine compounds, as well as vapor cabinets, were all found inadequate for sterilizing cystoscopes within one hour. Ten per cent formalin solution, used for fifteen minutes on a clean cystoscope, with all stopcocks open, proved to be eminently successful for killing all conventional organisms, including Mycobacterium tuberculosis.[7-9] The principal drawback was its capacity for irritating the skin of some of the personnel. It was necessary to wash it off in one of the more conventional fluids, in which the cystoscopes were then stored before use.

Incidence

The incidence of renal tuberculosis has at last shown some trend towards a decrease, for the last two years, after remaining remarkably constant at this research unit over the past twelve years, despite the advent and wide utilization of effective chemotherapy, including isoniazid, beginning about that time. Whether this reflects a vast reservoir of old cases or the fact that our unit is located in New York City, where there is a higher percentage of immigrants, or whether there will be an eventual drop-off in the numbers, remains to be seen. The clinical impression of many urologists that they are seeing less renal tuberculosis may only reflect the fact that they are being cured medically rather than coming to nephrectomy. It is a fact that even before the actual numbers of new cases decreased, the numbers of far advanced cavitary cases had decreased decidedly, the new cases consisting of moderately advanced (but distinctly cavitary) cases.[10]

The insidious nature of this disease can be judged by the fact that among the patients of this research unit, there were 25 physicians, 72% of whom showed advanced cavitary tuberculosis of the kidneys, a state of destruction that was achieved with so little disturbance to the patient that it did not lead to early diagnostic measures even in this more aware and knowledgeable group of patients. It has certainly been true that the disease had reached devastating proportions in both kidneys in many of these patients before it caused very much in the way of symptoms.[11] Many of the lesions were detected because pus cells were found in the urine at insurance examinations or because of the mildest backache, accompanied by slight pyuria.[12] The finding of ten pus cells per high-power field in a urine with a specific gravity of 1.015 is certainly compatible with renal tuberculosis, and it has been notable that among these patients, relapses were ordinarily accompanied by an increase in the number of pus cells.[13]

There has been recent widespread enthusiasm to adopt the utilization of the first-morning urine specimen instead of the twenty-four-hour urine accumulation for concentration and analysis for M. tuberculosis by culture and guinea-pig methods. To the best of my knowledge, this system has never been given adequate clinical trial on a comparative basis, where the two methods were used simultaneously on the same group of patients, at least in the United States. As far as can be determined, this attractive suggestion was made by Dr. Michael Kenney, as a result of nicely designed experiments in which artificially seeded specimens were used.[14] The advantages of smaller containers, quicker specimen collection and less opportunity for secondary contamination, in addition to Dr. Kenney's results, certainly argue strongly that this method might well be more practical than, and even superior to, the traditional twenty-four-hour urine collection. In a very small series of cases, the results have been found to be roughly parallel, but it will take a great many more cases before one can say whether there is any statistically significant difference between the two methods.

Although chromogenic acid-fast bacilli were recovered from the urine in 30 or 40 cases, there have been no well documented cases in which these organisms caused granulomatous renal disease, and most of the chromogens were thought to be contaminants.[15]

Antituberculosis treatment against genital tuberculosis is just as effective as against renal tuberculosis. It should be remembered that prostatic tuberculosis can be transmitted through the semen.[16]

Summary

Renal tuberculosis can be controlled by persistent, specific multiple-drug chemotherapy, based on drug-susceptibility information and abetted by adequate cystoscopic instrumentation to avoid stricturing. Triple-drug regimens used for a continuous period of two years are highly effective although the two-drug regimens may be equally effective if taken faithfully. Relapsing cases can be treated with different drugs, to which the organisms may still be susceptible. Excisional therapy is rarely, if ever, needed. Orally administered medications such as isoniazid, sodium PAS, ethambutol and cycloserine or ethionamide, as well as coverage with vitamin B_6, are usually adequate, even for retreatment, thus avoiding the unpleasantness and poor acceptability of injections with potentially toxic drugs such as streptomycin.

Patients with untreated urinary tuberculosis should be on precautions, and 10% formalin is the best agent for sterilizing cystoscopes contaminated with Mycobacterium tuberculosis. The incidence of urinary tuberculosis is not decreasing as rapidly as expected although the severity of the lesions does appear to be decreasing. The onset of the disease can be most insidious, as shown by the high incidence of advanced lesions among doctor patients.

REFERENCES

1. Segawa A and Reilly RJ: Unpublished data.
2. Reilly RJ: Unpublished data.
3. Gow JG: Genitourinary tuberculosis: study of 700 cases. Lancet 2:261-265, 1963.
4. Lattimer, JK and Reilly RJ: Present status of renal tuberculosis. Ann New York Acad Sc 106:96, 1963.
5. Lattimer JK, et al: Injections are no longer necessary in treatment of renal tuberculosis. Tr Am A Genito-Urin Surgeons J Urol 93:6, 735-738, 1965.
6. Vasquez G. and Lattimer JK: Danger to children of infection from exposure to urine containing tubercle bacilli. JAMA 171:29-33, 1959.
7. Lattimer, JK, Kenney M, Rosenblatt G, et all: Inadequate sterilization of cystoscopes. J Urol 76:197-199, 1956.
8. Wechsler H, Lattimer JK, Rosenblatt G, et al: Studies on sterilization of cystoscopes. Am Rev Tuberc 76:909-911, 1957.
9. Reilly RJ and Segawa A: Unpublished data.
10. Siegel J and Lattimer JK: Renal tuberculosis: has incidence of advanced lesions decreased in past two decades? J Urol 91:330, 1964.
11. Lattimer JK et al: Genitourinary tuberculosis: current status. In Transactions of the Twenty-second Research Conference in Pulmonary Diseases: Washington, D.C. Veteran's Administration. Department of Medicine and Surgery 46-51, 1963.
12. Wechsler H, Westfall M and Lattimer JK: Earliest signs and symptoms in 127 male patients with genitourinary tuberculosis. J Urol 83:801, 1960.
13. Lattimer JK and Kohen RJ: Renal tuberculosis. Am J Med 27:533, 1954.
14. Kenney M, Loeschel AB and Lovelock FJ: Urine cultures in tuberculosis. Am Rev Resp Dis 82:564, 1960.
15. Pellman CM: Significance of mycobacteria other than tubercle bacilli in urine. Am Rev Resp Dis 90:243, 1964.
16. Lattimer JK, Colmore HP. Sanger G, et al: Transmission of genitourinary tuberculosis via semen. Am Rev Tuberc 69:618-624, 1954.

※ ※ ※

LOCALIZATION OF URINARY TRACT INFECTION

• A proper epidemiologic and therapeutic approach to urinary tract infection requires accurate localization. Certain clinical, laboratory and instrumental tools assist in this procedure of localization.

WILLIAM BRUMFITT, M.D.

It has become apparent that localization of infection within the urinary tract has become increasingly important. When there is loin pain associated with tenderness and fever, there can be little doubt that infection of the renal parenchyma has occurred. In contrast with this situation, however, absence of typical symptoms and, indeed, total absence of symptoms, do not exclude the possibility of renal involvement.

Retrospective studies on children who have had urinary infection leave little doubt of the potential danger of this condition. In children it is well known that symptoms of urinary tract infection may be atypical, and there is frequently a delay in diagnosis. Reports from a number of centers make it apparent that delay in diagnosis of urinary tract and also of reflux, is associated with an increased incidence of scarring. Figure 1 shows the condition of the kidneys related to the age at the diagnosis of reflux.[1] It is evident that there is a much lower incidence of renal scarring in the younger age groups, whereas an increasing proportion of the older children with reflux have scarred kidneys. This probably reflects the longer exposure of the older child to this recurrent infection.

In this respect the work of Kunin, Deutscher and Paquin[2] is of great significance. They examined apparently normal schoolgirls between the ages of 5 and 19 years and showed that the prevalence of bacteriuria in girls was 1.2%. It should be stressed that this prevalence rate excluded children who had symptomatic infections and had therefore been treated before the survey was carried out. Most significant were the radiological findings of the asymptomatic children with bacteriuria because no fewer than 13.7% had caliectasis and 18.7%, reflux.

Before beginning a description of the methods for localization, it is necessary to stress that the urinary infection must be accurately diagnosed and that the sole criterion of urinary tract infection is the finding of significant bacteriuria. In our own experience it can be said that, with the exception of prostatitis, persistent infection within the urinary tract is almost always associated with a significant bacteriuria. It follows, therefore, that localization studies in the absence of significant bacteriuria are not worthwhile. To diagnose urinary infection the collection of an uncontaminated specimen of urine is essential. Both male and female patients must be given proper instructions together with the necessary materials to collect the specimen. Contamination is more likely to occur in the female, but satisfactory specimens can be obtained by the following procedure: the labia are separated and the vulva swabbed from front to back. With the labia still separated

Dr. Brumfitt, Ph.D., M.R.C.P., F.R.C. Path., is Consultant Clinical Pathologist, Edgware General Hospital; Consultant Bacteriologist, St. Mary's Hospital, London, W. 2; and Senior Lecturer in Bacteriology at the University of London.

33

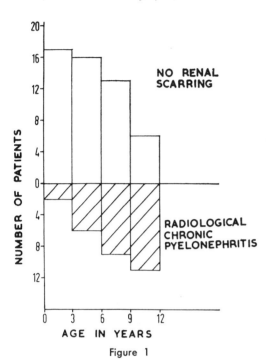

Figure 1

Results of I.V.P. in 80 children with reflux, relating the age at which reflux was diagnosed to the incidence of chronic pyelonephritis.

TABLE I

METHODS AVAILABLE FOR LOCALIZATION
OF INFECTION IN THE URINARY TRACT

Direct	Indirect
Urinary catheterization	Serum antibodies
Fairley technique	Urine concentration test
Renal biopsy	Urinary enzyme excretion
	Characteristics of urinary protein
	Prednisolone stimulation test

more). Counts within the range of 10^4 and 10^5 are equivocal and must be repeated. On repetition it will be found that most of these counts will move either into the range of infection (more than 10^5) or no infection (less than 10^3). The methods available for rapid and economical screening of urine specimens have been reviewed.[3]

Varieties of Urinary Infection

It is very important to appreciate that in defined groups of patients with bacteriuria the localization of the infection varies considerably. Thus in bacteriuria in pregnancy the chance of renal involvement is much greater than in patients with urethral syndrome who complain of frequency and dysuria. Nevertheless whenever the urine is infected, asymptomatic pyelonephritis will be present in a significant proportion of patients.

In the male, chronic prostatitis has long been recognized as a refractory condition frequently defying curative therapy, and infection in this organ must always be considered as the cause of recurrent bladder bacteriuria in the adult male.

Localization of Infection

The methods available for localization of infection are summarized in Table I. Kidney infection can be diagnosed directly by sampling ureteric urine, but distinction between upper and lower urinary infection using this method depends upon being able to wash out the bladder adequately, as well as other fac-

some urine is passed into the toilet, and then the disposable container provided is used to catch a midstream specimen. The urine should be sent to the laboratory within one hour or stored at 4°C; otherwise multiplication of a small number of bacteria present may invalidate the investigation. The diagnosis is made by quantitative counting, and the sole criterion of infection is a bacterial count of 10^5 or more. Whenever possible, all positive results should be confirmed by examination of a further urine specimen. The reason for this is that the confidence level of a single positive specimen is only 80%, whereas the finding of infection due to the same organism on a second occasion increases the confidence level to 95%. Within any population tested the vast majority of patients fall into those who are definitely not infected (that is to say, counts of 1,000 or less) or those who are definitely infected (that is to say, counts of 100,000 or

TABLE II
LOCALIZATION OF URINARY TRACT INFECTION BY BLADDER WASH-OUT

	Unilateral Ureteric Infection		Bilateral Ureteric Infection		Bladder Infection	
CASE NUMBER:	12	15	22	23	2	10
SEROTYPE	075	04	06	012	075	06
BLADDER						
*Bacteria	> 10^5	> 10^5	> 10^5	> 10^5	> 10^5	> 10^5
**WBC	327	247	264	84	28	750
RIGHT URETER						
*Bacteria	> 10^5	10^3	> 10^5	> 10^5	0	0
**WBC	490	197	0	28	0	820
LEFT URETER						
*Bacteria	0	0	> 10^5	> 10^5	0	0
**WBC	0	0	184	34	0	0
ANTIBODY TITER	1/1280	1/1280	1/2560	1/2560	1/160	1/1280
I.V.P.	CPN (Rt)	CPN (Rt)	poly-cystic kidneys	bilateral CPN	normal	CPN (Rt)

*Bacteria per ml
**WBC per cu mm

tors. Quantitative counts should therefore be made on the bladder wash-out fluid and no ureteric urine count regarded as significant unless it exceeds the bladder wash-out count by a factor of 10. In fact, differences are usually much greater. Removing bacteria from the bladder by wash-out is often especially difficult in cases with bilateral infection where ureteric counts are high. In such patients reinfection of the bladder contents presumably occurs continuously from above. Examples of uni- and bilateral ureteric urinary infection are shown in Table II. As in the case of bladder infection, pyuria may or may not be found to accompany infection of the ureteric urine.

It is most important to appreciate that in the ureter, where there is a continuous flow system, bacterial counts very much less than 10^5 are highly significant (e.g., case 15, Table II). Where there are hydronephrosis and ureteric dilatation in association with ureteric infection, bacterial counts may be very high because hydronephrosis of the ureter reduces the velocity of urine flow.

Examples of infection confined to the bladder are also shown in Table II. It should be noted that white cells may come from the bladder in the absence of upper urinary tract infec-tion and are therefore of no value in localiza-tion. The pyuria may persist for some time after eradication of infection from the ureter, and an example of this is shown in Case 10.

Neomycin Bladder Wash-out Test

We have used a modification of the test devised by Fairley[4] et al, the principle of which is shown in Figure 2. A Foley catheter is passed into the bladder and a specimen of bladder urine collected. The catheter is retained in position by inflating the balloon, and then 200 ml of neomycin solution at a strength of 0.1% is injected into the bladder and left in position for one hour. At the end of this time the bladder is washed out by 2 liters of water. A specimen of the wash-out fluid is collected to make sure that a bactericidal concentration of neomycin does not remain and that the bacteriuria has been eliminated. If urine specimens are then collected at ten minute intervals under conditions of mild diuresis, it is obvious that this urine will represent that being passed directly from the ureters. In this way, ureteric urine can be collected without the need to pass ureteric catheters. Some results of the neomycin bladder wash-out are shown in Table III. In the first example infection and pyuria are confined entirely to the bladder, whereas, in the second example,

TABLE III
LOCALIZATION OF URINARY TRACT INFECTION BY NEOMYCIN BLADDER WASH-OUT

		Bacterial count (per ml)		White cell count (per ml)	
		Case 1	Case 2	Case 1	Case 2
BLADDER URINE		>10^5	>10^5	27	1,155
WASHOUT FLUID		0	0	0	0
URETERIC URINE	10 MIN.	0	4x10^3	0	30
	20 MIN.	0	40x10^3	0	37
	30 MIN.	0	81x10^3	0	68
OSMOLALITY (m osmoles/kg H_2O)					
	SERUM	{ 855 883	{ 697 772		
	URINE	286	288		
SERUM ANTIBODY TITER		1/160	1/1280		

TABLE IV

CORRELATION OF REFLUX AND ANTIBODY
TITER IN CHILDREN

	Number of Children	RECIPROCAL OF ANTIBODY TITER	
		>320	<320
REFLUX	11	10	1
NO REFLUX	24	6	18
TOTAL	35	16	19

$$X^2 = 10.68 \quad : \quad p < 0.001$$

TABLE V

LEUCOCYTE EXCRETION IN NORMAL SUBJECTS

		Upper limit	Mean
Addis	(1926)	152,917	26,875
Rolfe	(1953)	206,600	28,200
Houghton and Pears	(1957)	196,000	87,700
Little	(1962)	109,000	24,930

where there is infection of the ureteric urine, bacteria rapidly reappear in the ten-minute collection specimens and there is a progressive rise in the bacterial count.

Indirect Techniques

It would, of course, be very useful to have a technique which would need only collection of specimens of urine and blood from the patient. We have developed such a technique based on the measurement of serum antibody against the organism causing the urinary infection.[5,6] It was found, by comparison with ureteric catheterization and obtaining kidney tissue from patients who had a partial nephrectomy, that when infection involved the kidney, the antibody titer exceeded a partic-

ular level. In contrast, when patients had no involvement of the renal parenchyma, the antibody titer was normal. This immunological method may be a better index of actual kidney tissue since involvement of the ureteric and pelvic urine does not necessarily mean renal parenchymal involvement. Figure 3 shows the result of the antibody titer test in patients with classical acute pyelonephritis where there was no doubt that the renal involvement had occurred. Serum samples were taken at intervals, and the highest titer was recorded. The results are shown by the open columns. The controls were patients who gave no history of urinary infection and whose urine was not infected at the time of examination. In the control patients no organism was available, and it was therefore necessary to test their serum against twelve of the most common O serotypes responsibile for urinary

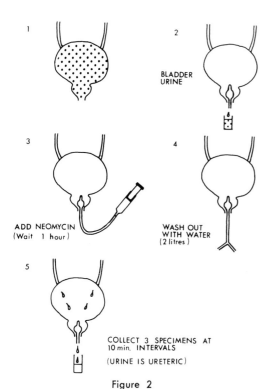

Figure 2

Fairley technique for localization of infection.

1. Bladder contains infected urine ($>10^5$ organisms per ml). The patient is told to empty the bladder completely and an M.S.U. is collected.
2. A Foley catheter is inserted and residual bladder urine collected and measured.
3. 50 ml. 0.1% neomycin sulphate solution is introduced into the bladder and left for 1 hour.
4. The bladder is repeatedly washed out with sterile water, using at least 2 litres. The bladder is then completely emptied and the last washing saved to test for residual neomycin.
5. Specimens of urine are collected at 10 minute intervals for at least 30 minutes.

infection, and to record the highest result. It can be seen that patients with renal involvement have high antibody titer whereas those without infection tested against the common O serotypes rarely exceed a titer of 1/160 and never 1/320. The method is a direct agglutination technique and is within the capacity of any properly equipped microbiological department. Thus, by estimating the titer it is possible to decide whether infection is confined to the bladder or involves kidney tissue (it must be remembered that in the male, prostatic involvement will also give a raised antibody titer even though no renal involvement is present). Serial readings can be of considerable help in confirming elimination of tissue infection. In patients with acute pyelonephritis a rise in titer occurs despite effective treatment, but following eradication of infection the titer falls to normal. In sharp contrast, patients with a persistent infection due to the same organism which resists eradication have a persistently raised antibody titer, as seen in Figure 4. In such cases where the infection is asymptomatic or not of abrupt onset, the titer is frequently raised when the patient is first seen and remains elevated. The dotted line (Figure 4) shows a case where infection was eradicated after an interval, and only then did the antibody titer fall. In children the test has been valuable, and Table IV shows the results of an investigation carried on in collaboration with Dr. Jean Smellie. It can be seen that where reflux is present, the antibody titer is almost invariably raised, whereas, if there is no reflux, the antibody titer is frequently not raised. Of course, the absence of reflux at any particular time does not eliminate the possibility of renal involvement. Nevertheless, the difference in antibody titer where reflux is present and where it is absent is significant.

| | Serum antibody titer | |
Bacteriuria in Pregnancy	Normal	Raised
No. treated	104	36
Cured	78 (75%)	20 (56%)
Frequency-dysuria syndrome		
No. treated	79	33
Cured	71 (90%)	19 (58%)

TABLE VI

EFFECT OF RENAL INVOLVEMENT ON THE RESULTS OF TREATMENT

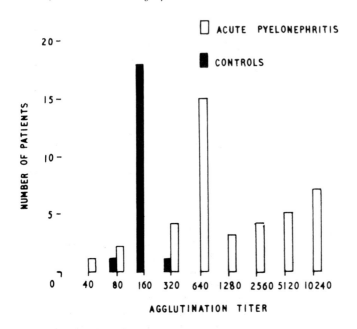

Figure 3

Comparison of serum antibody titer in 20 control patients and 41 patients with acute pyelonephritis.

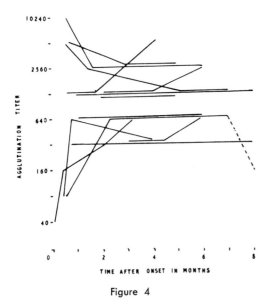

Figure 4

Persistence of high antibody titer in patients whose infections failed to respond to treatment. (Broken line indicates a fall in titer when therapy was ultimately successful.)

Urine Osmolality

Another test which enables distinction to be made between renal involvement and no renal involvement is estimation of the urine osmolality by means of osmometry. To carry out the test the patient was instructed to take no fluid from 12 noon but to eat a normal dry diet. The bladder was emptied at bedtime and the urine specimens collected the next day on waking and at 9 a.m. The urine osmolality was determined by depression to freezing point in a universal osmometer.

Ninety-six pregnant women were studied, and, of these, 63 had been shown to have significant bacteriuria on two successive occasions, while 33 were non-bacteriuric controls. Both groups studied were under identical conditions. The results are shown in Figure 5 where it can be seen that only one non-bacteriuric patient had a urinary osmolality below 750 milliosmoles/kg H_2O while in 32 (97%) the osmolality exceeded this value. In contrast, of the 63 bacteriuric women 19 (30%) showed values of less than 750 milli-

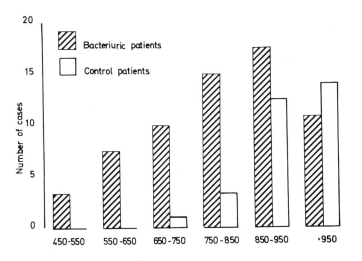

Figure 5

Results of urine concentration tests in pregnant bacteriuric patients and non-bacteriuric controls.

osmoles/kg H_2O. Thus the proportion of patients with bacteriuria in pregnancy who have renal involvement, as judged by impaired urine concentrating ability (30%), is similar to that found in pregnant women studied by Brumfitt and Percival[7] using the antibody technique (32%). The patients studied on both occasions were drawn from the same community and can, therefore, be regarded as being similar in many respects, including socio-economic status. Clearly the defective osmolality is not necessarily associated with chronic organic renal disease because, following successful treatment of the infection, we have observed the osmolality to return to normal.

Leucocyte Counts

We place great importance on the leucocyte counts, but they are no substitute for the tests mentioned in bacterial localization. The major difficulty is summarized in Table V where it is shown that there is a big variation between mean leucocyte excretion and the upper limit of leucocyte excretion. Furthermore, there is no method of determining the origin of leucocytes because techniques such as testing for the presence of "glitter cells" and the use of special stains have not proved to be effective in deciding whether the white cells originate from the bladder or from the upper urinary tract.

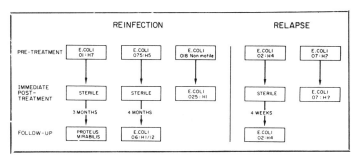

Figure 6

Infecting organisms isolated before and after treatment showing examples of reinfection and relapse. In the case of **E. coli** distinction can only be made by serotyping.

39

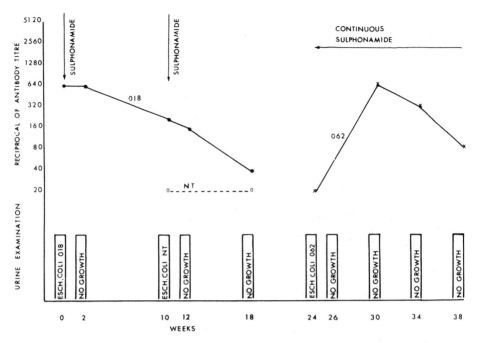

Figure 7 — Episodes of reinfection in a 14-year-old girl with a chronic renal lesion.

Other Methods

The other methods of localizing urinary infection, as listed in Table I, have not so far proved to be of practical value. The characteristics of urinary protein, urinary enzyme excretion and the prednisolone stimulation test are not, at the present time, widely used for purposes of localization.

Serotyping of E. Coli

If localization is to be used as a guide in the planning of treatment, serotyping of *E. coli* causing the infection is also important. *E. coli* is responsible for most domiciliary and so-called "spontaneous" urinary infections. If the urine becomes sterile after treatment, but later becomes infected by different organisms, such as *Proteus mirabilis* (Figure 6), reinfection by a new organism has obviously occurred. However, if the organism is still *E. coli*, it is impossible to know whether the same strain has persisted and relapse occurred, or whether the urine has become

reinfected from outside the urinary tract. Serotyping of the *E. coli* allows this distinction to be made. (Figure 6) A change in serotype group means reinfection, while the finding of the same serotype usually indicates relapse. It can be seen that both reinfection or relapse can be found immediately after treatment or during follow-up. However, in our experience relapse usually occurs in the six weeks following treatment,[8] and episodes after this interval are more likely to be due to reinfection. An example of reinfection is given below. (Figure 7)

A fourteen-year-old girl investigated for enuresis, was found to have an infection due to *E. coli* O 18, and a raised serum antibody titer indicated renal involvement. Treatment with sulfadimidine eradicated the infection, and the antibody titer subsequently fell to normal levels. There was a previous history of urinary infection, and radiology showed blunting of the right upper calyx, but no reflux was demonstrated. At ten weeks the

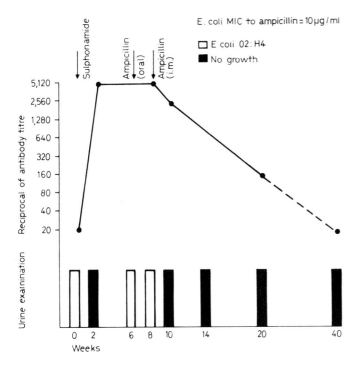

Figure 8

Relapse of infection in a 12-year-old girl with renal involvement but without radiological abnormality.

patient was asymptomatic, but the urine was found to be infected by a different strain of *E. coli* which could not be typed. The serum antibody against this organism was not increased. The infection again responded to sulfonamide, and six weeks later the urine was still uninfected. However, soon afterwards symptoms of lower urinary infection appeared, and *E. coli* O 62 was isolated from the urine. The raised antibody titer indicated that renal involvement had again occurred.

In view of the recurrent infection, evidence of renal involvement, and the presence of a chronic renal lesion, a course of sulfonamide was given and then continued in smaller doses. At the last examination the urine was uninfected and the antibody titer had fallen to normal.

This is an example not of failed chemotherapy but of the increased susceptibility to infection. Each episode of infection was eradicated, but reinfection by another strain of *E. coli* soon occurred.

Failure of therapy can be said to have occurred when the same organism reappears following treatment. This is illustrated by the following case. (Figure 8)

A girl aged twelve years, who had suffered from malaise and low grade fever, suddenly developed loin pain and fever of 101.6°. The urine was infected by *E. coli* O2: H4, and the subsequent rise of specific antibody indicated renal involvement. The patient was treated with sulfonamide, and the symptoms quickly disappeared. At follow-up the urine was sterile, but at six weeks an asymptomatic infection due to *E. coli* O2: H4 (the strain which caused the original infection) was found. This failed to respond to oral ampicillin at a dose of 500 mg 6 hourly. The reason for this failure is indicated in Figure 9, where it is seen that such therapy rarely gives serum levels (and possibly therefore tissue levels) which are adequate to eradicate certain infections involving the renal parenchyma. In contrast, intramuscular injection

41

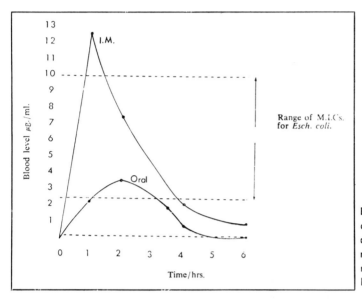

Figure 9

Blood levels of ampicillin obtained after administration of 500 mg by oral and intramuscular routes. The relationship of these levels to the range of M.I.C.s for "sensitive" **E. coli** is shown.

gives a much higher serum level. (Figure 9) The patient was therefore admitted to hospital and given a five-day course of intramuscular ampicillin, in order to obtain better blood levels — and presumably tissue levels. The urine became and remained sterile and the antibody titer fell to normal, reassuring us that the tissue involvement had been eradicated. Radiology of the urinary tract showed no abnormality. The patient has not been given prophylactic therapy, and the four year follow-up has shown no further episode of infection.

These examples indicate the great importance of not only determining the localization of the infection, but also of determining whether failure of treatment is due to failure of eradication or reinfection.

The Importance of Renal Involvement

In Table VI there is a substantial difference shown in the cure rate in asymptomatic bacteriuria in pregnancy, where the cure rate with conventional oral therapy is only 75%, and in the frequency-dysuria syndrome, common in women of childbearing age, where the cure rate is 90%. However, once renal involvement occurs, the cure rate is both lower and similar in the two groups.

Studies in Bacteriuria of Pregnancy

It is interesting to note that the localization of infection can be judged by follow-up studies of patients who have had a simple course of oral treatment. Our experience in 285 patients treated with sulfonamide shows that 74% responded and 26% failed. It is evident that treatment greatly decreases the risk of pyelonephritis in pregnancy, which can be reduced to very small levels if the treatment has been effective. Furthermore, the number of patients with bacteriuria who develop acute pyelonephritis, which is a serious complication of pregnancy, hazardous to mother and fetus, is approximately 25% in the untreated group, but, with treatment, the incidence can be reduced to between approximately 1.5% to 3%. Long term follow-up on patients who have had bacteriuria is also important. By the simple test of whether patients succeeded or failed to respond to sulfonamide, they can be divided into two different groups. The percentage with bacteriuria at follow-up, two to four years after the initial diagnosis, was 46% (22/48) in those who failed to respond to therapy but 19% (21/109) in those who responded. It should also be noted that the prevalence of infection in both groups is higher than that found in an unselected population of women of childbearing age where the prevalence is approximately 7%. This indicates that a substantial number of women in both groups are more susceptible to either continuous or recurrent urinary infection, so that long term follow-up of patients with bacteriuria in pregnancy is desirable. Radiology of patients with bacteriuria also shows that the same simple test of failing to respond to sulfonamide again divides patients very sharply into two groups. The failure group had abnormalities more frequently than the responding group, and the lesions tended to be more severe, 10 of the 11 patients with chronic pyelonephritis belonging to the group failing to respond.

Finally, in localizing infections the importance of the urological surgeon should not be ignored, for lesions within the bladder, such as a diverticulum, may well cause persistent or recurrent infections. In a non-draining diverticulum, bacteria reach a climax population (more than 10^9 per ml), and such populations are resistant to antimicrobial agents. Thus, the bladder urine can be easily sterilized by chemotherapy, but reinfection from urine within the diverticulum occurs each time chemotherapy is withdrawn.

In the male, recurrent infections always require detailed investigation to discover the reason, and lesions such as infection of the prostate and surgical lesions of the bladder must be borne in mind.

It is concluded, therefore, that although accurate diagnosis of urinary infection is still the keystone of treatment, it is also important to make an effort to localize infection, and it must be appreciated that symptoms alone are an inaccurate guide to the site of infection within the urinary tract.

REFERENCES

1. Smellie JM and Normand ICS: Clinical features and significance of urinary tract infections in children. Proc Roy Soc Med 59:415-417, 1966.
2. Kunin CM, Deutscher R and Paquin A Jr: Urinary tract infection in school children: an epidemiologic, clinical and laboratory study. Medicine (Balt) 43:91-130, 1964.
3. Brumfitt W: The detection and assessment of urinary infection. Recent Advances in Clinical Pathology, Dyke SC ed., London. Churchill, 19-33, 1968.
4. Fairley KF, Bond AA, Brown RB, et al: Simple test to determine the site of urinary tract infection. Lancet 2:427-428, 1967.
5. Brumfitt W and Percival A: Specific antibody response of patients with significant bacteriuria. Proc IInd Int Congr Nephr. Prague 1963, Excerpta Medica Foundation, Netherlands, 260-261, 1963.
6. Percival A, Brumfitt W and de Louvois J: Serum antibody levels as an indication of clinically inapparent pyelonephritis. Lancet 2:1027-1033, 1964.
7. Brumfitt W and Percival A: Serum antibody response as an indication of renal involvement in patients with significant bacteriuria. Progress in Pyelonephritis, Kass EH ed., Philadelphia, F A Davis, 118-128, 1965.
8. Williams JD, Brumfitt W, Leigh DA, et al: Eradication of bacteriuria in pregnancy by a short course of chemotherapy. Lancet 1:831-834, 1965.

PROPER URINE CULTURE TECHNIQUES IN INFANTS AND CHILDREN

• The diagnosis of urinary tract infection requires reliable and reproducible urine culture techniques. In the infant and small child, suprapubic bladder aspiration affords the best method for obtaining the urine specimen.

DAVID R. LINES, M.D.

Among the methods suggested for collecting urine for culture from infants and children are urethral catheterization, suprapubic aspiration and bag collection from either a grossly clean or surgically clean perineum. I propose to discuss these four methods of collection and the methods of examining the urine so collected to determine the presence of infection.

Firstly, let me point out the importance of detecting such infections early. Urinary infection is a significant cause of morbidity and mortality in childhood. Autopsy studies in childhood reveal an incidence of 1.6 to 2.0% of pyelonephritis.[1,2] In male children the age at which one is most likely to find a urinary infection is less than one month.

Secondly, let us consider the methods by which one may collect urine and their various virtues and disadvantages. As the young child or infant cannot void on demand, the practical policy to obtain naturally voided urine is to apply a bag to the perineum. This is usually done after careful surgical clean-up, usually using a combination of PhisoHex and Zephiran. Using such clean-up procedures in adult women where one has the advantage of obtaining a midstream specimen, up to 20% of urines have colony counts in the doubtful range.[3] One would presume that the application of a bag, which means the first few milliliters of urine are included, would lead to a higher rate of doubtful positives. The published figures comparing bag collection after surgical clean-up with either catheter collec-

tion or suprapubic aspiration in childhood show a contamination rate of 12 to 64%[4,5] with an increasing problem with younger age. This degree of uncertainty decreases with repeated samples, but repeated samples are not always possible in office practice.

Nor is the surgical clean-up procedure easily accomplished in a busy office practice, and it was this that prompted Dr. Randolph[6] to try the application of the bag to a grossly clean perineum. He found a contamination rate of only 3.5% using 10,000 colonies as a presumptive positive; this fell to 1½% with 100,000 colonies as the criterion. One possible criticism of this surprising result was that he checked his presumptive positives only against another bag count with surgical clean-up. However, if one presumes all of his positive cultures greater than 10,000 would have been proven not to be urinary infection by other means, his contamination rate would have been only 8%. Why did he find such a low rate of contamination? Does careful perineal clean-up actually increase the chance of contamination? The most likely reason I believe lies in the fact that he removed the bag and placed it in a refrigerator himself. This emphasizes the point that, no matter how careful the collection, immediate culture or refrigeration is necessary.

I would like to emphasize that in comparing contamination rates in naturally voided urines all investigators should compare their results with urine obtained either by urethral catheter or suprapubic aspiration which invariably shows lesser rates of infection and

Dr. Lines is with the University of Adelaide, Department of Child Health, The Adelaide Children's Hospital, Inc., Adelaide, Australia.

therefore, one presumes less likely to be contaminated.

The difficulties of catheterization especially in infants are known to you all and the dangers to most. The introduction of pathogenic bacteria can be reduced to a minimum as shown by Dr. Pryles' group in 1959.[7] However, in that study the catheterization was performed under anesthesia. In the conscious and therefore struggling child, the chance of infection rises remarkably.[8,9] In Dr. Pryles' study, sterile urine was obtained in 95.3% of cases who had suprapubic tap, while catheter urine was sterile in 59.5% when first few milliliters were examined and in 80.5% of cases if the second few milliliters were examined. All of the patients were considered to be free of infection, so here we have positive cultures in the face of these careful collection methods. If, however, one combines these methods of collection with colony count using 1000 colonies/ml as indicative of infection, one finds no positives with suprapubic aspiration and one case (2.5%) positive (presumably falsely so) in children older than three months who are anesthetized and catheterized after careful clean-up. I think it is a fair assumption that the contamination rate will rise when catheter collection is attempted in the conscious child. Thus when colony counting is used as the method of detection of infection, suprapubic aspiration or catheterization is much more accurate than bag collection.

Can we look at urine in any other way so that contamination is not a problem? The time-honored method of looking for pyuria is worthy of consideration.

Using 10 leucocytes/ml of urine (which approximates three pus cells/hpf) as a cut-off point, Mabeck[10] in Denmark was able to find pyuria in 95% of adult women with urinary tract infection. In children the rate of pyuria in urinary infections drops to 61%.[11] Thus if the detection of urinary infection relies on pyuria, it is likely more than one quarter of the children with infection will be missed. Perhaps more important is the fact that pyuria can have other causes than infection. In a review of the literature, the incidence of

pyuria in urines examined is 17.8%[12] whereas the incidence of significant bacteriuria is considered to be 5% or less.[13-15]

Chamber counting so that the pyuria is expressed as cells per milliliter is more accurate than counting cells/hpf, but a false positive rate three times as high as the true positive rate makes either method a screening test, and not a good screening test, in children where a quarter of the negatives are also false.

Leucocyte excretion rates further increase the accuracy of pyuria as an indicator of infection but are impossible to time and difficult to collect in uncooperative children.[10]

Gram staining of undiluted urine[16] and gram staining of the spun deposit[11] both show good correlation with bacterial counts, but neither is any better at ruling out contamination than colony count and both are less accurate.

The T T C and similar chemical tests for bacteriuria are again useful screening tests for pathogens with the exception of *Klebsiella*, which often does not register as a positive when it is the cause of infection. It does have the advantage of being able to be done by the person collecting the urine, but so does a colony count. In fact any person collecting a urine can easily plate out a loop full of urine far more easily than he can gram-stain or perform these chemical tests.

Other chemical tests, such as protein or blood in the urine, are positive in some urinary infections but are so variable as to be useless in helping one make a decision.[7] In fact one may as well look at a freshly voided urine and say, "If it is clear, it is unlikely to be infected; if cloudy, it may or may not be."

Thus we arrive at the conclusion that colony counting is the most reliable method of detecting urinary infection at our disposal. In turn the accuracy of colony counts depends on the method of collection. That suprapubic tap is the method that obtains least false positives is shown by numerous papers.[5,6,8]

Then why are we not using this method of collection? The objections are: 1. it is painful; 2. it is dangerous; 3. it may not obtain urine; 4. parents will consider it barbaric.

1. It does entail a certain amount of discomfort. That this is minimal is shown by Stamey's[18] ability to perform the aspiration in 2,500 adults, who reported that the passage of needle through the abdominal muscles was less painful than the subcutaneous local anesthesia. Thus without local anesthesia the procedure involves the same pain as an intramuscular injection, a mode of treatment likely to be chosen for the false positive urine infection. In fact it is probably less painful than the results of an ill-chosen clean-up fluid applied to the genitalia; alcohol-containing solutions are frequently used by inexperienced personnel.

2. Weathers and Wenzel[19] report three cases of perforation of organs other than bladder and allude to two others. In no case was any ill effect noted, and they concluded that in the child with a grossly distended abdomen, aspiration of urine is contraindicated. It is noteworthy that in the hospital where this occurred such bladder taps continue to be performed at a rate of about 40 per month. Although there may be other personal experience, no one else has felt compelled to report any complication of the procedure.

3. Failure to obtain urine can be avoided by ensuring that the bladder is palpable or percussable before aspiration. The full or partially full bladder is easily detected in the young child. If the bladder is not detected, one should wait (usually less than half an hour is necessary). This is not an indication for immediate bag collection because the child who has an empty bladder is unlikely to void spontaneously within half an hour.[6]

4. Parents will not consider suprapubic aspiration barbaric when educated regarding the procedure. It did not take much to convince patients that the dangers and discomfort of a penicillin injection were worthwhile. It should not take much to convince them that the bladder tap, which is less dangerous than any form of medication that one might incorrectly prescribe on the basis of any other collection, is worthwhile.

In conclusion, in the uncooperative child we know the most reliable method of urine collection, easier and faster than any other, is suprapubic aspiration.

REFERENCES

1. Neumann CG and Pryles CV: Pyelonephritis in infants and children. Am J Dis Child 104:215, 1962.
2. Butler AM and Lanman TH: NEJM 217:425, 1937.
3. Mabeck CE: Studies in urinary tract infection: II urinary tract infection due to coagulase-negative staphylococci. Acta Med Scand 186:39, 1969.
4. Nelson JD and Peters PC: Suprapubic aspiration of urine in premature and term infants. Pediatrics 36:132, 1965.
5. Newman CG, O'Neill P and Parker A: Pyuria in infancy and the role of suprapubic aspiration of urine in diagnosis of infection of urinary tract. Brit Med J 2:227, 1967.
6. Randolph MF and Greenfield M: The incidence of asymptomatic bacteriuria and pyuria in infancy. J of Pediatrics 65:57, 1964.
7. Pryles CV, Atkin MD, Morse TS, et al: Comparative bacteriologic study of urine obtained from children by percutaneous suprapubic aspiration of the bladder and by catheter. Pediatrics 24:983, 1959.
8. Helmholz HF and Millikin F: Personal communication.
9. Beeson PB: The case against the catheter. Am J Med 24:1, 1958.
10. Mabeck CE: Studies in urinary tract infections: IV. urinary leucocyte excretion in bacteriuria. Acta Med Scan 186:193, 1969.
11. Pryles CV and Eliot CR: Pyuria and bacteriuria in infants and children. Am J Dis Child 110:628, 1965.
12. Thysell H: Evaluation of chemical and microscopical methods for mass detection of bacteriuria. Acta Med Scand 185:393, 1969.
13. Larsson SO and Thysell H: Acta Med Scand 186:303, 1969.
14. Kass EH: Pyelonephritis and bacteriuria, a major problem in preventive medicine. Ann Intern Med 56:46, 1962.
15. Sallamander U and Ost C: Medicinsk Riksstamma, Stockholm, 1967.
16. Pryles CV and Steg N: Specimens of urine obtained from young girls by catheter versus voiding: a comparative study of bacterial cultures, gram stains and bacterial counts in paired specimens. Pediatrics 23:441, 1959.
17. Larsson SO and Thysell H: Acta Med Scand 186: 313, 1969.
18. Stamey TA, Govan DE and Palmer JM: The localization and treatment of urinary tract infections: the role of bactericidal urine levels as opposed to serum levels. Medicine (Baltimore) 44-1, 1965.
19. Weathers WT and Wenzl JE: Suprapubic aspiration of the bladder, perforation of a viscus other than the bladder. Am J Dis Child 117:590, 1969.

OXOLINIC ACID THERAPY OF RECURRENT URINARY TRACT INFECTIONS

- Oxolinic acid, a quinoline derivative, eradicated infection in a high percentage of patients with recurrent urinary tract infection. The incidence of side effects was high.

CLAIR E. COX, M.D.

Oxolinic acid, an organic acid, is the second of two quinoline derivatives which exhibit antibacterial and pharmacologic[1-4] properties consistent with those required for agents used in the therapy of urinary infections. The first of these two organic acids, nalidixic acid, was shown to be effective in the treatment of urinary tract infections.[5-7] On the other hand, as experience with the drug accumulated, it has been suggested that the usefulness of nalidixic acid may, to some extent, be limited by its tendency to rapidly evoke bacterial resistance,[6,7] the not uncommon occurrence of gram-positive superinfection during nalidixic acid therapy,[5] and the relatively high incidence of side effects which occur with nalidixic acid administration.

Clinical experience with oxolinic acid is limited; however, two reports have indicated that it is effective for urinary-tract infections.[7,8] It is suggested by one of these studies[7] that oxolinic acid is less prone than nalidixic acid to "evoke highly resistant mutant bacteria." Oxolinic acid is known to be more potent on a weight basis[1,7] than nalidixic acid and therefore, a smaller dose of medication is theoretically required for similar infectious processes. This paper describes our experience with oxolinic acid in the treatment of 67 patients with recurrent urinary tract infections.

Dr. Cox is with the Department of Surgery, Division of Urology, Bowman Gray School of Medicine of Wake Forest University, Winston-Salem, North Carolina.

Supported-in-part by the Warner-Lambert Research Institute, Morris Plains, N. J.

METHODS

Laboratory Studies

All bacterial isolates were identified by standard procedures and tested by the single disc technique[9] to oxolinic acid discs of the following concentrations: 0.5 mcg, 1.0 mcg, 2.0 mcg and 5.0 mcg. The minimal inhibitory concentration (MIC) and minimal bactericidal concentration (MBC) of each clinical isolate were determined by a tube dilution technique as previously described.[10] A standardized inoculum of approximately 10^5 organisms was used. Final concentrations of oxolinic acid were 25, 12.5, 6.25, 3.12, 1.56, 0.78, and 0.39 mcg/ml.

Serologic grouping for the determination of the somatic (0) antigen was performed on all *E. coli* isolates.

Clinical Studies

Sixty-seven outpatients, attending the private urological clinic of the Bowman Gray School of Medicine, were placed into a study to evaluate the efficacy of oxolinic acid in the therapy of urinary infection. Each patient had a urinary tract infection at the time of initial treatment with oxolinic acid as indicated by a pretreatment urine culture demonstrating 10^5 or greater bacteria per ml of urine. All but three of these 67 patients had a history (usually confirmed by our records) of recurrent episodes of urinary infection. Forty-three of the patients were female and 24 male. The age range was 16 to 65 with a mean age of 44.

49

OXOLINIC ACID #1
RESULTS
M.I.C.

	No. Isolates	Cumulative % isolates sensitive µg./ml. oxolinic acid					
		≤ 0.39	0.78	1.56	3.1	6.25	12.5
E. coli	42 (42)*	60	79	95			
P. mirabilis	25 (7)	56	73	92			
Indole pos proteus	25 (2)	51	71	89			
Coliforms	25 (2)	53	68	91			
Kleb. –aerobacter	25 (7)	31	47	64	81	93	
Pseudomonas	10 (0)						20

* figures in ( ) indicate isolates from study patients

TABLE 1: Cumulative percent of 142 urinary pathogens sensitive to increasing concentrations of oxolinic acid.

At the time of therapy with oxolinic acid 41 patients were diagnosed as having cystitis, 18 prostatitis, and eight pyelonephritis. Prior infections of the urinary tract had occurred on an average of between five and six times in these 67 patients.

Oxolinic acid was administered in a dose of 750 mg twice daily for 28 days. In the event that side effects occurred, the dosage was to be reduced to 500 mg twice daily. Prior to and immediately following treatment a complete blood count, urinalysis, BUN, and SGOT were performed on all patients. Urinalyses, urine cultures, and patient evaluations were carried out on the seventh, fourteenth, and final therapy day; and, in addition, the same studies were performed after completion of therapy at monthly intervals for three months.

RESULTS

Laboratory Studies

Table 1 shows the cumulative percent of 152 urinary pathogens susceptible to increasing concentrations of oxolinic acid determined by the tube dilution technique in broth. It should be noted that 60 of these gram-negative organisms were obtained from the study patients and the remaining 92 from additional patients with urinary infections. With the ex-

ception of *Klebsiella-Enterobacter* isolates, 89 to 95% of the Enterobacteriaceae were inhibited by 1.56 mcg/ml or less of oxolinic acid. Although *Klebsiella-Enterobacter* strains were less susceptible, 93% were inhibited by 6.25 mcg/ml, an amount of oxolinic acid well below urinary concentrations of the drug and a level of drug which can be attained in the serum.[11] *Pseudomonas* strains were uniformly resistant to oxolinic acid. When compared to similar tube-dilution studies with nalidixic acid, by us[5] and others,[6] it is clear that oxolinic and nalidixic acid have a similar spectrum of activity, but it is equally evident that oxolinic acid is more potent on a weight basis.

The zone of inhibition about discs containing 0.5 mcg, 1.0 mcg, 2.0 mcg, and 5.0 mcg was measured for the isolates recovered from the study patients and compared with the MIC as measured by tube dilution. These results are shown in Figure 1. Separation into resistant and sensitive populations and consistency between disc zones and MIC's were best achieved with the 2 and 5 mcg discs. This is especially true if the staphylococcal isolates are removed.

Minimal bactericidal concentrations, although not illustrated here, were most com-

OXOLINIC ACID #1
BACTERIOLOGIC RESULTS

	No. Patients	Therapy 1–49 days*			Patients at risk	Recurrence	
		Eradicated	Persistent	Superinfection		0–28 days	28–84 days
E. coli	41	37	3	1	37	3 (1)**	7 (1)
Klebsiella-aerobacter	7	5	2	0	5	1 (1)	2
Proteus mirabilis	6	5	0	1	5	0	2 (1)
Indole pos. proteus	2	2	0	0	2	1	0
Staph. albus	6	6	0	0	6	1	1
Other gram negatives	3	3	0	0	3	1	2
mixed infections	2	2	0	0	2	1	0
Totals	67	60	5	2	60	22 (4)	

* mean 26 days
** figures in ( ) indicate recurrences due to relapse, remainder due to re-infection

TABLE 2: Bacteriologic results in 67 patients treated with oxolinic acid.

monly equal to the MIC, occasionally one tube higher, and rarely more than one tube above the MIC.

Clinical Studies

Although a 28-day course of therapy was planned in all cases, actual therapy ranged from one to 49 days with a mean therapy duration of 26 days. Six patients were treated from one to seven days, five from eight to 14 days, seven from 15 to 26 days, 47 from 27 to 33 days and two from 40 to 49 days. The principal reason for changes in therapeutic duration was the occurrence of side reactions. Side effects were noted in 18 of the 67 (26.8%) study patients. The dosage was reduced from 750 mg twice daily to 500 mg twice daily in 14 of these 18 patients, but, in general, side effects occurred at a similar rate with either dosage. If side effects were present with a dose of 750 mg twice daily, most often they persisted, although slightly less prominent, with a 500 mg twice daily dose. Three of the 18 patients experiencing reactions continued therapy for the entire 28 days; however, therapy was discontinued 27 to seven days prior to planned termination of therapy in the remaining 15 patients. One of the 18 patients developed an apparent allergic cutaneous rash which cleared promptly with discontinuation of therapy on the 13th day of treatment. Reactions in the remaining 17 patients were equally distributed between the gastrointestinal and central nervous system. Gastrointestinal reactions were primarily nausea and vomiting and were considered mild in five instances, moderately severe in ten and severe in one instance. Central nervous system reactions were mainly those which could be broadly categorized as excitability: restlessness, insomnia, nervousness, etc. These were considered mild in nine cases and moderately severe in six cases.

Symptomatic response to therapy was prompt and, in general, paralleled the bacteriologic response as noted below. Of interest are the several patients in whom therapy was terminated prior to 28 days but yet in whom the infection was eradicated.

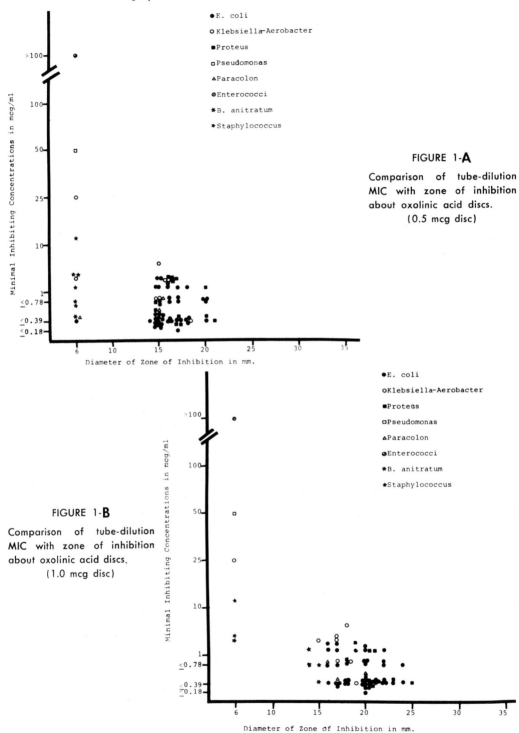

FIGURE 1-**A**

Comparison of tube-dilution MIC with zone of inhibition about oxolinic acid discs. (0.5 mcg disc)

FIGURE 1-**B**

Comparison of tube-dilution MIC with zone of inhibition about oxolinic acid discs. (1.0 mcg disc)

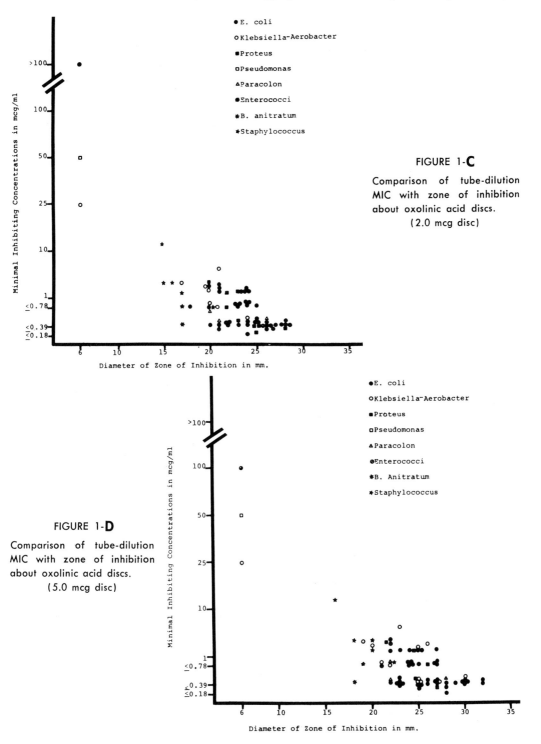

FIGURE 1-**C**

Comparison of tube-dilution MIC with zone of inhibition about oxolinic acid discs.
(2.0 mcg disc)

FIGURE 1-**D**

Comparison of tube-dilution MIC with zone of inhibition about oxolinic acid discs.
(5.0 mcg disc)

Complete blood counts, urinalysis, BUN and SGOT were performed on all patients prior to and following therapy. In no instance were there noted any significant changes in these studies.

Bacteriologic Response

The bacteriologic results for the patients are summarized in Table 2. Urinary infection was eradicated in 60 of the 67 (89.5%) study patients. The infection was persistent in five instances, and superinfection occurred in two patients. Follow-up results (Table 3) reveal a recurrence of infection (two relapse and six re-infection) in eight of the 60 patients during the first follow-up month. Recurrence of infection was noted in an additional 14 (two relapse and 12 re-infection) patients during the subsequent two follow-up months. Overall recurrence of infection was noted in 22 (four relapse and 18 re-infection) of the 60 patients at risk during the three months following oxolinic acid therapy.

Results of serotyping for the somatic (0) antigen were used to aid in the differentiation between relapse and re-infection.

Comments

The *in vitro* bacteriologic results described in this report indicate that oxolinic acid is highly effective against *E. coli, Proteus mirabilis*, indole positive proteus, intermediate coliforms, and to a slightly less extent, *Klebsiella-Enterobacter*. These *in vitro* results correlated well with the clinical studies in which urinary infection was eradicated from 60 of the 67 patients treated with oxolinic acid. Of interest were six patients in the study with urinary infection due to *Staphylococcus albus*. Although the oxolinic acid disc zones (Figure 1) for these staphylococci were somewhat smaller than the gram-negative zones, the MIC's were 3.1 mcg/ml or less in five of the six cases. Therefore, the six patients were treated with oxolinic acid, and in all instances the infections were eradicated. However, in our experience the majority of staphylococci and all enterococci are resistant to oxolinic acid.

The therapeutic results (89.5% bacterial eradication) described in this report are considerably better than those of D'Alessio et al,[8] who used a lower dose and shorter duration of therapy, but are comparable to those of Ronald et al,[6] who noted a 74% cure rate in 23 patients treated with oxolinic acid with a dose of 1000 mg twice daily for 14 days.

Infection persisted in five of the 67 patients treated with oxolinic acid. Four of the five persistent organisms demonstrated posttreatment resistance to oxolinic acid, and the MIC of the fifth increased from 0.39 mcg/ml to 6.25 mcg/ml posttreatment. Resistance emergence at this rate (5/67) does not seem unusually high and is consistent with the observations of Ronald et al,[6] who noted clinically significant resistant mutants in only one of 23 patients. On the other hand, Dr. D'Alessio et al,[8] treating with a dose of 500 mg twice daily, noted a considerably higher rate of resistance emergence. Therefore, both with regard to the prospect of bacterial eradication as well as minimizing the emergence of resistant mutants, this study and that of Ronald et al[6] both strongly favor a dose of oxolinic acid of at least 1.5 grams daily and for a minimum of 14 days.

The recurrence rate in this study was eight of 60 patients during the first follow-up month and 22 of 60 during the entire three month follow-up. This rather low recurrence rate (36.6%) is impressive for several reasons: (1) 64 of the 67 study patients had histories of recurrent urinary infection, (2) the follow-up period of three months in this report is longer than follow-up periods in similar reports, and (3) most (18 of 22) of the recurrences were due to re-infection.

Overall 38 of 67 (67 less seven persistent infections, less 22 recurrences) patients in this three-month study were cured with respect to eradication of and continued freedom from urinary infection. These satisfactory bacteriologic results are slightly minimized by the rather high occurrence (26.8%) of reactions to oxolinic acid. On the other hand, no toxicity was noted, and the gastrointestinal and CNS reactions were promptly reversed by discontinuation of therapy.

Summary

Oxolinic acid was administered to 67 patients with recurrent infectious disease of the urinary tract. Although reactions to oxolinic acid occurred in 26.8% of the patients, urinary infection was eradicated from 89.5%. Emergence of resistance was relatively minimal, and a recurrence rate during three months of follow-up was only 36.6%.

REFERENCES

1. Turner FJ, Ringel SM, Martin JF, et al: Oxolinic acid, a new synthetic antimicrobial agent. I. In vitro and in vivo activity. Antimicrobial Agents and Chemotherapy, 1967, p 475-479.
2. Ringel SM, Turner FJ, Lindo FL, et al: Oxolinic acid, as new synthetic antimicrobial agent. II. Bactericidal rate and resistence development. Antimicrobial Agents and Chemotherapy, 1967, p 480-485.
3. Ringel SM, Turner FJ, Roemer S, et al: Oxolinic acid, a new synthetic antimicrobial agent. III. Concentrations in serum, urine and renal tissue. Antimicrobial Agents and Chemotherapy, 1967, p 486-489.
4. McChesney EW, Froelich EJ, Leshner GY, et al: Absorption, excretion, and metabolism of a new antibacterial agent, nalidixic acid. Toxicology and Applied Pharmacology 6:292-309, 1964.
5. Harrison LH and Cox CE: Bacteriologic and Pharmacodynamic Aspects of Nalidixic Acid. To be published by the Journal of Urology.
6. Ronald AR, Tuck M and Petersdorf RG: A critical evaluation of nalidixic acid in urinary tract infections. NEJM 275:1081-1088, 1966.
7. Atlas E, Clark H, Silverblatt F, et al: Nalidixic acid and oxolinic acid in the treatment of cronic bacteriuria. Ann Intern Med 70:713-721, 1969.
8. D'Alessio DJ, Olexy WM and Jackson GG: Oxolinic acid treatment of urinary tract infections. Antimicrobial Agents and Chemotherapy 490-496, 1967.
9. Bauer AW, Kirby WMM, Sherris JC, et al: Antibiotic susceptibility testing by a standardized single disc method. Amer J Clin Path 45:493-496, 1966.
10. Cox CE: Gentamicin, a new aminoglycoside antibiotic: Clinical and laboratory studies in urinary tract infection. J Inf Dis 119:486-491, 1969.
11. Cox CE: Oxolinic acid therapyof urinary tract infection patients with impaired renal function: Clinical and laboratory results. Unpublished data, presented at the 7th Annual Infectious Disease Symposium, May 5-8, 1970, Wilmington, Delaware.

MINOCYCLINE IN THE TREATMENT OF URINARY TRACT INFECTIONS

● A new tetracycline has been evaluated in the treatment of acute and chronic urinary tract infections. In this limited study, there was good clinical efficacy with minimal side effects.

WILLIAM J. HOLLOWAY, M.D.

Minocycline (7-dimethylamino-6-deoxy-6-demethyltetracycline) is a new semisynthetic tetracycline which has a broad antibacterial spectrum. It is effective *in vitro* against many gram-positive and gram-negative bacteria including tetracycline-resistant staphylococci. Several reports[1-3] in the literature attest to its *in vitro* effectiveness, suggesting that it is the most effective tetracycline now available for clinical use. Animal studies have been reported[4] showing its effectiveness *in vivo*, but there are few reports[3] in the clinical literature of the use of minocycline in the treatment of human infections.

This study describes the use of minocycline in the treatment of patients with acute and chronic urinary tract infections. As a corollary to this study, minocycline was evaluated in the treatment of patients with bacterial respiratory infections, and these results will be reported separately.

Material and Methods

Forty-two patients with urinary tract infections were selected at the Wilmington Medical Center and the Brandywine Medical Center for inclusion in this study. Most of the patients with chronic urinary tract infection were from the Pyelonephritis Clinic of the Wilmington Medical Center, while the majority of the patients with acute urinary tract infection were from the population of the Brandywine Medical Center. There were 29 female and 13 male patients ranging in age from 16 to 85 with a median age of 54. The 42 patients fell into the following clinical categories: acute cystitis, nine patients; chronic cystitis, seven patients; acute pyelonephritis, six patients; chronic pyelonephritis, 17 patients and asymptomatic bacteriuria, three patients.

Minocycline (supplied by Lederle Laboratories*) was administered in a dosage of 100 mg every 12 hours following an initial loading dose of 200 mg. In some instances, in prolonged therapy, the dosage was reduced to 100 mg given once daily. The duration of therapy ranged from ten days to 18 months.

Patients included in the study were monitored by the following parameters before, during and following minocycline therapy: complete blood count, urinalysis, blood urea nitrogen, serum creatinine, total bilirubin, alkaline phosphatase and serum glutamic oxaloacetic transaminase. Serum and urine specimens were obtained from a representative number of patients for measurement of antibiotic and antibacterial levels.

Pathogens isolated from patients in this study were tested for susceptibility to minocycline by the disc-agar diffusion and test tube dilution techniques. In addition, during the annual antibiotic screen in 1968 and 1969, representative strains of gram-negative and gram-

Dr. Holloway is Director, Infectious Disease Research Laboratory, Wilmington Medical Center, Wilmington, Delaware.

* Courtesy of Hugh MacDonald, M.D.

57

TABLE No. 1

RESULTS OF THERAPY — URINARY TRACT INFECTIONS

Type	Success	Number of Patients		
		Qualified Success	Failure	Indeterminate
Acute Cystitis	8			1
Chronic Cystitis	2		5	
Acute Pyelonephritis	6			
Chronic Pyelonephritis	9	2	4	2
Asymptomatic Bacteriuria	3			
TOTAL	28	2	9	3
		GRAND TOTAL	42	

positive pathogens were tested for susceptibility to minocycline using a standardized disc-agar diffusion technique.

Results of Therapy

Table No. 1 lists the results of therapy in these 42 patients treated with minocycline. The results were categorized as success, qualified success, failure and indeterminate. Patients considered to have a qualified success were those in whom chronic infection was satisfactorily controlled with resultant abacteriuria during maintenance therapy with minocycline but who relapsed when therapy was discontinued. In patients in whom it was impossible to assess the role that the antibiotic played in the final outcome of the infection, the result was considered indeterminate. Successes and failures need no explanation. As can be seen in the table, 27 patients experienced a successful result with an additional three patients being considered as qualified successes. Nine patients failed to respond to therapy with minocycline while in three patients, the results were considered indeterminate.

Acute Cystitis

Eight of the nine patients suffering from acute cystitis showed a prompt satisfactory response to minocycline therapy, while in one patient the result was considered indeterminate. In this patient, the cystitis followed an indwelling foley catheter and was due to a strain of enterococcus. Prompt symptomatic relief and urine sterilization resulted from the use of minocycline, but side effects prompted discontinuing the antibiotic on the third day and the results were considered indeterminate. *Escherichia coli* was the infecting organism in all eight patients with acute cystitis who responded favorably to minocycline therapy.

Chronic Cystitis

Five of seven patients suffering from chronic cystitis failed to respond to minocycline therapy. In three of these five failures, the infecting organism was a *Klebsiella* species while two patients were infected with a *Proteus* species. One patient with chronic cystitis due to *Escherichia coli* had a qualified success in that throughout six months of therapy (minocycline 100 mg daily), urine sterility was maintained, but on cessation of minocycline therapy, relapse with a resistant strain of *Escherichia coli* occurred. One patient with chronic cystitis due to a *Klebsiella* species received minocycline therapy for six weeks with relief of symptoms and a sterile urine for six months following cessation of therapy.

Acute Pyelonephritis

All six patients who suffered from acute pyelonephritis showed a satisfactory response to minocycline therapy. In each instance, therapy was continued for a minimum of two weeks. The infecting organism was an *Escherichia coli* in three instances and *Enterobacter*

TABLE No. 2

MINOCYCLINE SERUM LEVELS

(22 patients)

Time	Range
One Hour	1.3 to 4.5 mcg/ml
Three Hours	1.2 to 3.5 mcg/ml
Five Hours	1.1 to 2.5 mcg/ml
Eleven Hours	0.6 to 2.3 mcg/ml

DOSE: 100 mg every twelve hours

in two instances; one patient was infected with an enterococcus. All of these infecting organisms were sensitive to minocycline *in vitro*.

Chronic Pyelonephritis

The response to therapy in chronic pyelonephritis was not as gratifying as in the acute infections, though several of these cases responded to long-term therapy with minocycline. All 17 patients with chronic pyelonephritis received a minimum of six weeks of minocycline therapy, and in some instances, therapy was continued as long as 18 months. The infecting organisms in the nine patients with chronic pyelonephritis who had a successful outcome were as follows: *Escherichia coli*, four cases; mixed infection with *Klebsiella* and *Escherichia coli*, one case; and one case each of *Citrobacter*, *Klebsiella*, *Pseudomonas* and *Enterobacter*. The two patients with chronic pyelonephritis who were considered as qualified successes were infected with strains of the *Klebsiella* species. These patients had failed to respond to other modalities of therapy and became asymptomatic and abacteriuric during eight weeks of minocycline therapy, but relapsed with the same organism following treatment. Two of the four patients with chronic pyelonephritis who failed to respond to minocyline therapy were infected with strains of *Pseudomonas* species, while one patient was infected with *Klebsiella* and another with *Escherichia coli*. In both instances where the results were considered indeterminate, there had been significant reduction in the

bacterial colony count (*Proteus* and enterococcus), but it became necessary to discontinue therapy because of gastrointestinal side effects.

Asymptomatic Bacteriuria

Two patients with asymptomatic bacteriuria due to *Escherichia coli* and one patient infected with a *Klebsiella* were treated for six weeks with minocycline therapy and in each instance had a satisfactory response, with subsequent sterile urine cultures over a six-month follow-up period.

Side Effects

All 42 patients in this study were interviewed frequently to detect any side effects due to the antibiotic. Six patients reported gastrointestinal side effects manifested by nausea and vomiting in five instances and diarrhea in one patient. The diarrhea disappeared on continuation of therapy, and in two of the five patients with nausea and vomiting, this likewise subsided though therapy was continued. However, in three instances, the continued nausea required cessation of therapy, though in two of these three patients, therapy had been continued for a period of six weeks before nausea required discontinuation of minocycline.

The period of this study included two summers without evidence of photosensitivity. The patients were monitored by the above mentioned parameters, and the only instance of laboratory abnormality was an eosinophilia (9%) in one patient during the third week of therapy.

Laboratory Data

Table No. 2 lists minocycline serum levels in 22 patients, drawn at varying intervals following multiple dosing of minocycline, 100 mg every 12 hours. At one hour, the serum level ranged from 1.3 to 4.5 mcg/ml, while at 11 hours there was still a measurable level of minocycline in the serum ranging from 0.6 to 2.3 mcg/ml. Serum antibacterial levels performed on these same specimens revealed inhibition of the infecting organism in concentrations of 1:4 or better in a majority of the 20 specimens tested.

Ten strains of each	Minocycline	Tetracyline	Doxycycline
	(average concentration in mcg/ml)		
Pseudomonas species	38.8	67.5	80.0
Escherichia coli	3.05	42.8	15.6
Klebsiella species	7.97	19.8	15.9
Enterobacter species	16.2	17.1	21.0
Proteus species	70.0	100	100

TABLE No. 3

COMPARISON OF IN VITRO EFFECTIVENESS OF MINOCYCLINE, TETRACYCLINE & DOXYCYCLINE

Table No. 3 compares the *in vitro* effectiveness of minocycline with tetracycline and doxycycline against ten strains of each of five common, gram-negative urinary pathogens. It can be seen that minocycline compares favorably and is as good as or better than the other tetracyclines against all of these common pathogens.

Extensive *in vitro* evaluation of minocycline has been carried out during the annual antibiotic disc susceptibility testing carried out at the Wilmington Medical Center. Both the 5 and 30 mcg minocycline discs have been included in various portions of this study utilizing a well standardized disc-agar diffusion technique. The 5 mcg minocycline disc showed a satisfactory inhibitive zone (greater than 15 mm) against 98% of 200 clinical isolates of *Staphylococcus aureus*. In addition, the 5 mcg disc was effective against 68% of the strains of *Escherichia coli*, 57% of the strains of *Klebsiella*, and 25% of the strains of enterococcus. The 30 mcg disc showed a satisfactory zone (greater than 15 mm) against 91% of the strains of *Klebsiella*, 95% of the strains of *Escherichia coli*, 72% of the strains of *Proteus* but only 10% of the strains of *Pseudomonas aeruginosa*. When testing the clinical isolates from patients in this study, there appeared to be a satisfactory correlation between the disc-agar diffusion and the test-tube dilution technique.

Discussion

While minocycline is active against tetracycline-resistant strains of staphylococci, the development of several new antistaphylococcal antibiotics makes it less likely that this agent will find clinical usefulness in the treatment of staphylococcal infections. However, this tetracycline does have a broad antibacterial spectrum with good *in vitro* and *in vivo* activity. In agreement with other reports[1,3] in the medical literature, our *in vitro* data suggest a slight advantage for minocycline over the other available tetracyclines in the medical literature, and we agree with other workers[2] that the *in vitro* susceptibility testing with tetracyclines can be greatly affected by variations of technique.

In this limited study, minocycline appears to be effective in the treatment of acute urinary tract infections due to tetracycline-sensitive organisms. As one would expect, the results in chronic urinary tract infection are less satisfactory. However, since more than 50% of the patients with chronic infection in our study had a successful outcome from minocycline therapy, further clinical trials with this antibiotic are indicated. No attempt was made to compare minocycline in a controlled manner with any of the other available tetracyclines. However, our past experience[5,6] with the evaluation of other tetracyclines in the Pyelonephritis Clinic would suggest to us that minocycline is as good as any of the other tetracycline agents available for clinical use.

Summary

Minocycline, a new tetracycline antibiotic, showed satisfactory *in vitro* effectiveness against a wide range of gram-positive and gram-negative microorganisms. This antibiotic was utilized in the Pyelonephritis Clinic in the treatment of patients with acute and chronic urinary tract infections. In 16 patients with acute urinary tract infections, there were 15 successful responses while one patient had an indeterminate response. Fifteen of 26 patients with chronic urinary infections showed a successful response to therapy, while in nine patients there was a failure to show a significant response, and in two patients the response was considered indeterminate.

The usual dose of minocycline was 200 mg daily in two divided doses, with therapy being continued over a period of 14 days to 18 months. In a few selected patients, long-term therapy was continued with 100 mg of minocycline given once daily. The antibiotic was well tolerated with occasional gastrointestinal side effects.

REFERENCES

1. Steigbigel NH, Reed CW and Finland M: Susceptibility of common pathogenic bacteria to seven tetracycline antibiotics in vitro. Amer Journ of Med Sciences 255:179-195, 1968.
2. Washington JA II, Yu PKW and Martin JM: In vitro antibacterial activity of minocycline and effect of agar medium utilized in its susceptibility testing. Applied Microbiology 19: 259, 1970.
3. Frisk AR and Tunevall G: Clinical evaluation of minocycline. Antimicrobial Agents and Chemotherapy 335-339, 1969.
4. Redin GS: Antibacterial activity in mice of minocycline, a new tetracycline. Antimicrobial Agents and Chemotherapy 371-376, 1967.
5. Holloway WJ, Kahlbaugh RA and Scott EG: Methacycline in the treatment of urinary tract infections. Del Med Journ 39:245-249, 1967.
6. Holloway WJ, Furlong JH and Scott EG: Doxcycline in the treatment of infections of the urinary tract. Journ of Urology 102:249-252, 1969.

CEPHALEXIN IN THE TREATMENT OF URINARY TRACT INFECTIONS

• Cephalexin is almost completely absorbed after oral administration producing excellent blood and urine levels. This antibiotic shows considerable promise in the treatment of acute and chronic infection of the urinary system.

Leo B. Hogan, M.D.

The cephalosporin antibiotics, cephalothin and cephaloridine, have received extensive clinical usage in the past few years. They have been reported to produce excellent results in various infections caused by gram-positive and gram-negative microorganisms.[1-4] The major disadvantage of these cephalosporins has been the necessity for their administration by the parenteral route.

Cephaloglycin, the first oral cephalosporin-C derivative to be made available, has been used extensively in clinical trials for the treatment of urinary tract infection.[5-8] This antibiotic will soon be available for clinical usage. Cephaloglycin produces satisfactory urine levels for the treatment of urinary tract infections, but blood levels with this antibiotic are not adequate for the treatment of systemic infections. With cephaloglycin, there has been a high incidence of gastrointestinal side effects, most notably diarrhea.

Cephalexin, the second cephalosporin derivative available for oral administration, has now had extensive clinical trials in the treatment of a variety of infections.[9,10] While this antibiotic seems to be less effective *in vitro* than the other cephalosporins against the common pathogens, the high blood and urine levels obtained after oral administration make this an interesting compound for further clinical trial. Also, cephalexin is so completely absorbed from the gastrointestinal tract that

Dr. Hogan is an Internist in private practice in Wilmington.

the incidence of diarrhea with this cephalosporin antibiotic should be considerably less than that experienced with cephaloglycin. The expectation that this antibiotic would be highly effective in the treatment of urinary tract infections prompted the current study.

Material and Methods

Patients with acute and chronic urinary tract infection were selected from the medical and surgical services of the Wilmington Medical Center, the Pyelonephritis Clinic of the Wilmington Medical Center, and the private outpatient population of the Brandywine Medical Center. Forty-four patients ranging in age from 8 to 78 years were selected for inclusion in the study. All patients in the study had positive urine cultures with plate counts greater than 10^5 organisms per ml. Eighteen of the 44 patients had chronic pyelonephritis while four had acute pyelonephritis. Nine patients had acute cystitis, eight had chronic cystitis, and five had chronic unclassified urinary tract infection. The patients selected were infected with a variety of urinary pathogens including *Escherichia coli* (21 cases), *Klebsiella* (ten cases), *Proteus* species (11 cases), *Enterobacter* (one case) and atypical coliform (one case). Toxicity studies included a hemogram, chemistry 12 profile (SMA 12) and urinalysis obtained before, at one week intervals during, and after therapy. When possible, blood and urine specimens were obtained for antibacterial and antibiotic assay. Appropriate pre- and post-treatment cultures were obtained in each instance and at one- or two-week intervals in patients on prolonged therapy. The susceptibility of the infecting organisms to cephalexin was determined by the two-fold serial tube dilution technique, and all strains were tested by the disc agar diffusion technique utilizing 30 mcg discs of cephalexin as well as all of the other antibiotics used in our routine susceptibility testing.

Cephalexin was supplied by the Eli Lilly Company as capsules containing 250 mg of the drug and in sterile vials of 20 mg for laboratory investigation. The cephalexin was administered by mouth in doses of 250-500 mg every six hours.

Results

Thirty-two of the 44 patients receiving cephalexin therapy experienced a satisfactory response to this antibiotic. Nine patients were considered treatment failures, and in three instances the response was indeterminate. Six of the nine patients with treatment failures had the original organism eradicated and relapsed with a secondary pathogen. In the remaining three instances of failure, the original pathogen was not eradicated. Six of the nine treatment failures had chronic infection (five chronic pyelonephritis, one chronic unclassified urinary tract infection), and all six had been followed for a long period of time in the Pyelonephritis Clinic. Most of these patients had failed to respond previously to other methods of treatment of chronic urinary tract infection.

In the six instances in which failure was associated with relapse with a different infecting pathogen, the new pathogen was cephalexin-resistant, the original infecting organism having been cephalexin-sensitive. In the three instances where failure was due to inability of the antibiotic to eradicate the original infecting organism, this organism was cephalexin sensitive suggesting that factors other than antibiotic failure were responsible for treatment failure.

The follow-up period in these patients showing a satisfactory response to cephalexin

has varied from one to twelve months. Because of the easy accessibility of the majority of these patients, long term follow-up should be possible and can be reported at a later date.

One of the four patients with acute pyelonephritis deserves special mention. This was a 78-year-old female patient with acute pyelonephritis complicated by sepsis, and *Escherichia coli* was isolated from her blood stream. Cephalexin 750 mg was given by mouth on a four-hour schedule for five days, at which time it was changed to 500 mg every six hours for an additional five days. She subsequently was given 250 mg every six hours for two weeks giving a total treatment period of 24 days. She showed an excellent clinical response, and three months after cessation of cephalexin therapy, the urine culture was sterile. Six months after cessation of therapy, an *Escherichia coli* was again isolated from the urine though the patient was clinically well at the time. Because of her diabetes and the severe sepsis that she originally suffered, she was placed on long term cephalexin therapy, and now 18 months after her initial illness, she remains free of symptoms with a sterile urine culture.

Side Effects

Three of the 44 patients treated with cephalexin in this study experienced significant side effects (7%). In two instances, the side effects were severe enough to require cessation of therapy. One young female patient developed a vaginitis with marked pruritis and swelling which was severe enough to require cessation of therapy. An additional patient developed a generalized pruritis, and while there was no evidence of rash, the symptoms were severe enough to prompt cessation of cephalexin therapy. The only patients who developed gastrointestinal side effects experienced mild diarrhea which the attending physicians felt might not have been due to the cephalexin.

Ten of the 44 patients in this study showed mild alterations in their toxicity studies which may have been drug related. They were as follows: three patients showed mild elevation of the serum glutamic oxaloacetic transaminase level: in two of these patients, there was a transient elevation with a return to normal levels during the course of therapy while in the third patient, the transaminase returned to normal level after cessation of therapy. Three patients showed a relative eosinophilia of 6% or greater while on cephalexin therapy, and one patient developed a mild leukopenia (3400 WBC/cu mm) with a normal differential. All counts returned to normal levels within a few days after stopping cephalexin. In three instances, patients had transient glycosuria while receiving cephalexin therapy. These patients were not known to have diabetes mellitus, and this revelation prompted glucose tolerance tests in two of the three patients after cephalexin therapy. Both tests were completely normal.

Antibiotic Assay

Blood and urine for assay were obtained from a representative number of patients receiving 250-500 mg of cephalexin every six hours. The average blood level in 19 patients, one hour after dosing on the initial day of therapy was 21 mcg/ml; after five or more days of therapy, the average cephalexin blood level one hour after dosing in nine patients was 27 mcg/ml.

Random urine specimens were obtained in 15 patients for determination of cephalexin levels. These ranged from 50 mcg/ml to 3250 mcg/ml with an average level of 938 mcg/ml.

Summary

Forty-four patients with acute and chronic urinary tract infections were treated with cephalexin in a dosage of 250 or 500 mg at six-hour intervals. A satisfactory response was achieved in 72% of the patients treated. Most of the failures were in patients with chronic urinary tract infection who had been attending Pyelonephritis Clinic for a number of years and had failed previously to respond to other modalities of therapy. Cephalexin produced therapeutic blood and urine concentrations which far exceeded the *in vitro* bactericidal inhibitory concentrations of the antibiotic for the pathogens treated. Since these blood and urine levels can be obtained after oral administration of this antibiotic, it has obvious advantages over previous types of cephalosporin antibiotics available for clinical use.

While there was no attempt to carry out a controlled study comparing the side effects with cephalexin with those due to cephaloglycin, it appears that cephalexin produces a lower incidence of gastrointestinal side effects than the other oral cephalosporin derivative. It appears that further investigation is indicated to evaluate the proper role of this new antibiotic agent in the treatment of infectious diseases.

REFERENCES

1. Kaplan K, Reisberg BE and Weinstein L: Cephaloridine: antimicrobial activity and pharmacologic behavior. Am J Med Sci 253:667-674, 1967.
2. Griffith RS and Black HR: Cephalothin — a new antibiotic. J Am Med Assoc 189:823-828, 1964.
3. Holloway WJ and Scott EG: Clinical experience with cephalothin in the treatment of severe infections. Antimicrobial Agents and Chemotherapy 215-219, 1964.
4. Holloway WJ and Scott EG: Clinical experience with cephaloridine. Antimicrobial Agents and Chemotherapy 916-921, 1965.
5. Hogan LB, Holloway WJ and Jakubowitch RA: Clinical experience with cephaloglycin. Antimicrobial Agents and Chemotherapy 624-629, 1967.
6. Johnson WD, Applestein JM and Kaye D: Cephaloglycin: clinical and laboratory experience with an orally administered cephalosporin. JAMA 206:2698-2702, 1968.
7. Kunin CM and Brandt D: Comparative studies of ampicillin, cephalothin and a new cephalosporin derivative, cephaloglycin. Am J Med Sci 255:196-201, 1968.
8. Landes RR, Melnick I, Fletcher A, et al: Cephaloglycin: a new orally effective antibiotic for urinary tract infections. J of Urology 102:246-248, 1969.
9. Wick WE: Cephalexin, a new orally absorbed cephalosporin antibiotic. Appl Microbiol 15: 765-769, 1967.
10. Foord RD, Dash CH and Johnson SE: Cephalexin, an early appraisal. Progress in Antimicrobial and Anticancer Chemotherapy 1:705, 1970.

THE SIGNIFICANCE OF THE INTESTINAL MICROFLORA

• Alterations in the normal bowel flora contribute to a number of clinical syndromes and disease entities. A better understanding of the ecologic balance between these microorganisms is mandatory.

Sydney M. Finegold, M.D.

Normal Gastrointestinal Flora

Although presently used techniques do not allow for recovery of all intestinal organisms which may be visualized directly, considerable progress has been made in recent years in documenting the normal bacterial flora at various levels in the gastrointestinal tract. The stomach normally has very small numbers (less than 10^3/ml) of organisms.[1,2] The organisms seen include yeast, viridans streptococci and lactobacilli. Counts tend to be higher in gastric samples with higher pH's, particularly above pH 4.0. Counts rise to 10^5/ml and the flora is more varied following a meal; the pre-meal level is reached again in 30-45 minutes following the meal.[1]

In the upper small intestine, the flora is relatively simple and counts are usually in the range of 10^3 to 10^5.[1,2] The upper small bowel flora is made up primarily of gram-positive aerobic organisms, although small numbers of gram-negative anaerobic bacilli may be seen as well. Again, after a meal the counts increase and the flora becomes more complex, but most of the newly acquired organisms disappear within one and a half hours of the meal.[1]

As one progresses from the upper small bowel to the ileum, the flora increases in number and type. In the terminal ileum, Bacteroides and Bifidobacterium predominate, with coliforms in slightly smaller numbers.[1,2] In feces, the two dominant organisms are *Bacteroides fragilis* and Bifidobacterium, both being present at levels of 10^{10} to 10^{11}/gm of wet feces.[1,3] These two organisms account for more than 99% of the cultivable flora. Coliforms are the next most commonly isolated group, normally being present at a level of 10^6-10^7/gm and thus accounting for less than 0.1% of the total bacterial population. Other anaerobes found in feces include Sphaerophorus, *Bacteroides melaninogenicus*, Fusobacterium, Eubacterium, Clostridium and anaerobic cocci of various types. Lactobacillus is an aerobic or microaerophilic gram-positive bacillus found in about 50% of people, with mean counts (when present) of 10^7/gm. Other aerobic or facultative forms found include various types of enterococci and streptococci of the viridans type.

The flora of the small intestine may be much more profuse in the presence of pathology of various types, particularly obstruction.

Effect of Antimicrobial Drugs on Bowel Flora

Although many of the studies on the effect of antimicrobial compounds on the bowel flora are inadequate because of lack of proper anaerobic techniques and for other reasons, a considerable amount of information is at hand concerning these effects. A summary of the effect of various antimicrobial drugs on the normal bowel flora has recently been prepared.[4] Interest along this line has centered primarily about the possibility of staphylococcal enterocolitis as a complication of antibiotic

Dr. Finegold is Chief, Infectious Disease Section; Associate Chief, Medical Service, Wadsworth Veterans Hospital; and Professor of Medicine, Department of Medicine, UCLA School of Medicine, Los Angeles, California.

therapy. The likelihood that organisms other than staphylococci may be important in this regard is discussed later in this manuscript. Modification of the normal flora may also interfere significantly with certain physiologic processes related to bowel flora, to be noted subsequently.

Changes in the bowel flora may also be induced selectively by antibiotics so as to determine the relative importance of various segments of the flora in certain physiologic functions and in various pathophysiologic states. For example, one can eliminate anaerobic bacteria with little or no change in aerobic flora by the use of oral lincomycin or one can eliminate aerobes with retention of most of the anaerobic flora by the use of oral kanamycin or related drugs. Oral polymycin eliminates *E. coli* and oral bacitracin may be used to decrease or eliminate streptococci and clostridia. It is important that one always does appropriate quantitative cultures to determine exactly what effect was produced in the particular patient under study since the results are not always predictable.

Effect of Intestinal Flora on Antimicrobial Drugs

Although much has been done regarding the effect of antimicrobial agents on the intestinal flora, it has not been generally appreciated that the reverse (effect of intestinal flora on antimicrobial agents) may be very important.[5] Two examples of this type of activity are the hydrolysis of succinyl- and phthalyl-sulfathiazole to the active drug, sulfathiazole, and the effect of the bowel flora on sulfadimethoxine (Madribon-Roche) which is normally excreted in the biliary tract as the glucuronide. The bowel flora deconjugates the glucuronide thus liberating free drug which is then reabsorbed. This enterohepatic circulation may account for the long duration of activity of this drug.

Importance of Normal Flora

Although the intestinal flora undoubtedly plays an extremely important role in the body's nutrition and physiology, comparatively little is known about this activity. We do know that *E. coli* and *Bacteroides fragilis* are capable of synthesizing vitamin K. Under

certain circumstances, vitamin K production by intestinal bacteria may be important to the host. Since *B. fragilis* greatly outnumbers *E. coli* in the normal intestinal flora, it is reasonable to assume that *B. fragilis* is much more important in this regard.[6]

Bile acids play a very important role in fat absorption, bile formation, and regulation of cholesterol metabolism.[7] Intestinal bacteria modify bile acids in various ways including deconjugation of the attached glycine and taurine, dehydroxylation of the primary bile acids (cholic and chenodeoxycholic acids) to form the secondary bile acids (deoxycholic and lithocholic acids) and a number of other changes not all of which have been well characterized. The significance of some of the transformation products remains to be determined as well. In any case, it is known that the action of intestinal bacteria on bile acids is important for their conservation by means of enterohepatic circulation. Deconjugation of bile salts may be carried out by a number of bacteria, those of importance in the intestinal tract being *Bacteroides fragilis*, various species of Sphaerophorus, Bifidobacterium, other gram-positive anaerobic bacilli and, among the aerobic organisms, *Streptococcus faecalis*.[8,9] Dehydroxylation of bile acids is carried out by various gram-positive anaerobic bacilli and, to a limited extent, by some strains of *B. fragilis*, *Veillonella* and some aerobes.[8] Inasmuch as deoxycholic acid is the major bile acid found in feces, it is surprising that the dominant members of the fecal flora cannot be shown to have significant capacity to dehydroxylate cholic acid.

The conversion of bilirubin to urobilinogen is carried out by intestinal flora and may be interfered with by administration of certain antibiotics, such as chlortetracycline. However, the organisms in the normal bowel flora responsible for this conversion have not been identified.

It has been shown that neomycin in small doses may decrease the serum cholesterol and the cholesterol pool in the body.[10] It can also be shown that with neomycin therapy this type bile acid excretion is increased, but that whereas there is normal deconjugation of bile acids there is no conversion of cholic acid to deoxycholic acid. Whether neomycin, in this circumstance, acts by means of an effect on the intestinal bacterial flora or not remains to be determined.

The normal bacterial flora of the intestinal tract is certainly important in terms of a variety of infections which may arise secondary to perforation of the bowel, strangulation, obstruction by carcinoma or other mechanisms, or following bowel surgery. *B. fragilis* is one of the major organisms likely to be found in such infections, along with coliforms and enterococci; other anaerobes may be involved as well.

The possibility that intestinal bacteria may serve directly or indirectly as a source for re-infection in patients with recurrent urinary tract infection has been considered by many workers, and there is increasing evidence accumulating to indicate that this may be a fact.

The normal flora of the bowel constitutes one of our most important defense mechanisms, a fact that is not generally appreciated. In this connection, the excellent studies of Bohnhoff, Miller and Martin[11] are of interest. These workers showed that mice are rendered much more susceptible to experimental Salmonella infection after treatment with oral streptomycin which reduces the counts of *Bacteroides* in the mouse intestine. Salmonella infection in man may have been exacerbated or activated by ampicillin and oxytetracycline.[12,13] Dubos and Schedler[14] have shown that NCS mice, raised in isolation, have a predominance of lactobacilli in their intestinal flora. These animals are different from conventional mice in having a better early growth rate, the ability to grow on an imbalanced diet, resistance to lethal action of endotoxin and greater susceptibility to certain experimental systemic bacterial infections.

Diarrhea Following Antibiotic Therapy

In general, it has been considered that diarrhea and other lower gastrointestinal symptoms relating to antibiotic therapy are the result of a direct irritant effect of the drug. However, there are many ways in which

alteration of the bacterial flora might explain these types of symptoms. Staphylococcal enterocolitis is a well-established entity which may result from a change in bowel flora related to antibiotic therapy.[15] Salmonella infection following antibiotic therapy has just been discussed. There seems to be good evidence that, at least in infants, severe and even fatal diarrhea may be caused by *Klebsiella* and *Pseudomonas* and perhaps *Proteus*. There are other organisms known to be causes of diarrhea, the proliferation of which might be favored by antimicrobial agents, but there are no documented cases of such superinfection on record. Included in this group would be such organisms as enteropathogenic *E. coli*, *Shigella*, *Edwardsiella* and *Yersinia*. In addition, the normal flora of the bowel includes enterococci and *Clostridium*, both of which have been described as causes of food poisoning. An increase in counts of either of these types of organisms, or perhaps selection of certain strains with special capabilities of causing enteritis, might account for diarrhea following antibiotic therapy. Indeed, we have some tentative evidence[16] suggesting the possibility that significant increase in counts of enterococci may account for the diarrhea with lincomycin therapy — a sort of endogenous food poisoning.

We are becoming aware of a number of specific ways in which changes in bowel flora might account for diarrhea. These might be related to the types of changes which have just been discussed or perhaps to more subtle changes or rearrangements of the normal flora of the bowel. For example, several amines are considered to be toxic. Twenty-one of 26 infants with gastroenteritis of "unknown etiology" had phenylethylamine in their stools.[17] Phenylethylamine is produced by enterococci. Increased amounts of lactic acid or certain volatile fatty acids, all end products of metabolism of certain intestinal organisms, might account for some cases of diarrhea related to antibiotic therapy.[18] The dihydroxy bile salts, deoxycholate and chenodeoxycholate, have the property of inhibiting the reabsorption of sodium and water.[19] Conversion of bile salts by intestinal bacteria has already been referred to. Still another bile acid, lithocholic acid, induces inflammatory reactions when present in the free form. Lithocholic acid normally is found in the intestine in the sulfated form which is non-toxic,[19] but it is possible that certain intestinal bacteria might be capable of splitting off the sulfate portion of the molecule. Finally, studies of fecal fat in patients with steatorrhea have revealed the presence of a number of non-dietary fatty acids, principally 10-hydroxy-stearic acid.[20] Since these acids are not present in any dietary fats, they are presumably synthesized in the gut by bacteria. Long chain hydroxy acids are not found often in oils and fats, but are particularly evident in resins and oils used as cathartics.

It follows from what has been said that it is extremely important to choose an agent which modifies the normal flora least from among several that might otherwise be suitable for treatment of a given infection.

Intestinal "Sterilization"

While there are theoretical advantages to decreasing or eliminating bacteria from the intestinal tract prior to bowel surgery, and while many surgeons still prefer to attempt to do this, there is increasing evidence to suggest that this type of practice may not actually be beneficial and that there are certain hazards which may attend it. For example, a double blind study evaluating preoperative intestinal sterilization carried out at our hospital[21,22] indicated that patients getting either oral neomycin or oral kanamycin as preoperative bowel preparation had a significant incidence of *Staphylococcus aureus* in their feces and a significant percentage of postoperative infection of various types due to this same organism. On the other hand, placebo-treated patients had no *S. aureus* in the stool and no infections with this organism. In the antibiotic-treated group, there was also some overgrowth of other organisms such as *Klebsiella* and *Pseudomonas* in the feces which would be potentially harmful. Furthermore, the one thing which one might hope to accomplish with such preoperative bowel preparation — elimination or reduction of infections due to such elements of normal flora as *E. coli* and Bacteroides — was not accom-

plished. In addition, there is some evidence[23] to indicate that patients who have had antibiotic therapy prior to bowel surgery for malignancy are more likely to develop recurrence of cancer at the suture line subsequently.

It is well known that patients with hepatic coma or pre-coma often respond well to antimicrobial therapy such as oral neomycin. This is thought to be related to the reduction of intestinal flora which produces ammonia, although it is likely that other compounds may play a role in this clinical picture as well. While most workers have thought of urease-producing organisms as being the major offenders in this situation, the possibility remains that organisms capable of producing ammonia by deamination are important. Furthermore, information is needed as to just which organisms in the intestinal tract are the prime offenders, regardless of the mechanism.

Miscellaneous Conditions in Which Intestinal Flora Is Important

The "blind loop syndrome" and related types of malabsorption having in common bacterial overgrowth in the upper small bowel may be treated effectively with appropriate antimicrobial agents. It has already been pointed out that anaerobic bacteria are particularly important in deconjugating bile acids in the small bowel. Such deconjugation interferes with proper micelle formation and therefore leads to improper fat absorption and steatorrhea. The use of lincomycin in a patient with the blind loop syndrome, in whom both gram-negative anaerobic bacilli and coliforms were isolated from afferent loop contents, indicated that the offending organisms in this particular patient were the anaerobic gram-negative bacilli.[24] There is reason to believe that anaerobes are a major cause of this type of problem in general. Other situations in which overgrowth of bacteria in the small bowel may account for malabsorption, since a response may be obtained to antibiotic therapy, include tropical sprue, diabetic neuropathy and scleroderma.

Although specific pathogens have not been implicated in "traveler's diarrhea," the fact that this may be prevented with certain antimicrobial drugs indicates that there is some specific alteration of the flora which should be detectable with appropriate studies.

Some cases of so-called functional diarrhea may really represent abnormal alteration of flora without presence of a specific pathogen.

Herman's syndrome (lymphonodular hyperplasia of the small bowel with immunoglobulin A deficiency) may have malabsorption related to either bacterial overgrowth in the small bowel or giardiasis or both. We have had occasion to study one patient with this syndrome and found that the upper small bowel contents had a high count of organisms commonly found in the oral flora.

Patients with ileal bypass for obesity sometimes develop significant hepatic damage as a result of the operation. While there are no specific studies on this point, it is conceivable that this may be related to alterations of bacterial flora, perhaps in turn resulting in overproduction of lithocholic acid or some other toxic product. Lithocholic acid does induce bile duct proliferation,[19] and excessive production of sodium taurolithocholate by intestinal bacteria can cause a syndrome of cholestasis.[7]

Feeding of lithocholic acid to rats leads to gallstones formed of insoluble calcium salts of either free or glycine-conjugated lithocholic acid or a hydroxylated lithocholic acid. Calcium glycolithocholic stones might occur in human beings who had bacterial overgrowth of the small intestine.[25] Lithocholic acid would be produced by dehydroxylation of chenodeoxycholic acid in the small bowel. This might also cause liver damage. Feeding of bile salts to humans may lead to a proportionately greater increase in phospholipid than in cholesterol in the bile and a proportionately greater increase in both of these compounds than in bile acids.[26] This type of response suggests the possibility that a lack of adequate bile acid production and/or bile acid reabsorption might be an important factor contributing to the presence of insufficient amounts of bile acids and phospholipid to solubilize biliary cholesterol.

Finally, we come to the interesting possibility that intestinal bacteria may play a role in intestinal cancer. Large bowel malignancies are more prevalent in developed than in under-developed countries, Japan representing a notable exception. Immigrants from areas with a low incidence of bowel cancer tend to show the same high incidence of this cancer as the local populace.[27,28] Changes in diet may be very important in this regard, and diet is known to affect the intestinal bacterial flora.[28] It is interesting in this connection to note that degradation of bile salts is an important metabolic activity of intestinal bacteria and that it is possible using various bacteria in the laboratory to convert deoxycholate into 20-methylcholanthrene, a very potent carcinogen.

Summary

We have outlined the make-up of the normal intestinal flora and discussed briefly the effect of antimicrobial drugs on bowel flora and the effect of the bowel flora on antimicrobial drugs. We have given a number of examples of how the normal flora of the bowel is or may be important to the host. We have discussed possible mechanisms for diarrhea following antibiotic therapy and have considered the matters of preoperative bowel flora depletion and of the use of antimicrobial drugs in hepatic coma. Finally, we have briefly considered a variety of pathologic conditions in which bacteria are known to be important or in which they may play a role.

REFERENCES

1. Drasar BS, Shiner M and McLeod GM: Studies on the intestinal flora. I. The bacterial flora of the gastrointestinal tract in healthy and achlorhydric persons. Gastroenterology 56:71-79, 1969.
2. Finegold SM: Intestinal bacteria — the role they play in normal physiology, pathologic physiology, and infection. Calif Med 110:455-459, 1969.
3. Finegold SM and Miller LG: Normal fecal flora of adult humans. Bacteriol Proc 93, 1968.
4. Finegold SM: Interaction of antimicrobial therapy and intestinal flora. Am J Clin Nutrition, In Press.
5. Peattle JR: The role of the gut flora in drug toxicity. Dissertation submitted for Diploma of Chelsea College in Biopharmaceutics, 1969.
6. Gibbons RJ and Engle LP: Vitamin K compounds in bacteria that are obligate anaerobes. Science 146:1307-1309, 1964.
7. Javitt NB: Clinical aspects of bile acid metabolism. Schweiz Med Wochenschr 8:269-272, 1968.
8. Hill MJ and Drasar BS: Degradation of bile salts by human intestinal bacteria. Gut 9:22-27, 1968.
9. Shimada K, Bricknell KS and Finegold SM: Deconjugation of bile acids by intestinal bacteria: review of literature and additional studies. J Inf Dis 119:273-281, 1969.
10. Samuel P, Holtzman CM, Meilman E, et al: Effect of neomycin on exchangeable pools of cholesterol in the steady state. J Clin Inv 47:1806-1818, 1968.
11. Bohnhoff M, Miller CP and Martin WR: Resistance of the mouse's intestinal tract to experimental salmonella infection. I. Factors which interfere with the initiation of infection by oral inoculation. J Exp Med 120:805-816, 1964.

12. Rosenthal SL: Exacerbation of salmonella enteritis due to ampicillin. NEJM 280:147-148, 1969.
13. Finger D and Wood WB Jr: The apparent activation of salmonella enteritis by oxytetracycline. Am J Med 18:839-841, 1955.
14. Dubos R and Schaedler RW: Some biological effects of the digestive flora. Am J Med Sci 224:265-271, 1962.
15. Finegold SM and Gaylor DW: Enterocolitis due to phage type 54 staphylococci resistant to kanamycin, neomycin, paromomycin and chloramphenicol. NEJM 263:1110-1116, 1960.
16. Finegold SM, Harada NE and Miller LG: Lincomycin: activity versus anaerobes and effect on normal human fecal flora. Antimicrobial Agents and Chemotherapy, 1965, Amer Soc for Microbiol. Ann Arbor, Michigan, 659-667, 1966.
17. Bachrach U, Sterk VV, Gery I, et al: Volatile amines in stools of infants suffering from gastroenteritis. Am J Hyg 72:1-5, 1960.
18. Weijers HA and van de Kamer JA: Alteration of intestinal bacterial flora as a cause of diarrhea. Nutrit Abst and Rev 35:591-604, 1965.
19. Palmer RH: The significance of bile salts metabolism. Hospital Practice 4:71-79, 1969.
20. James AT, Webb JPW and Kellock TD: Fatty acids in fecal lipids. Biochem J 78:333-339, 1961.
21. Gaylor DW, Clarke JS, Kudinoff Z, et al: Preoperative bowel "sterilization" — a double-blind study comparing kanamycin, nemycin and placebo. Antimicrobial Agents Annual — New York, Plenum Press, Inc. 392-403, 1960.
22. Gordon HE, Gaylor DW, Richmond DM, et al: Operations on the colon — The role of antibiotics in preoperative preparation. Calif Med 103:243-246, 1965.
23. Herter FP and Slanetz CA Jr: Preoperative intestinal preparation in relation to the subsequent development of cancer at the suture line. Surg Gynecol Obst 127:49-56, 1968.
24. Polter DE, Boyle JD, Miller LG, et al: Anaerobic bacteria as cause of the blind loop syndrome. A case report with observations on response to antibacterial agents. Gastroenterology 54:1148-1154, 1968.
25. Small DM: Gallstones. NEJM 279:588-593, 1968.
26. Swell I and Bell CC Jr: Influence of bile acids on biliary lipid excretion in man. Implication in gallstone formation. Am J Dig Dis 13:1077-1080, 1968.
27. Wynder EL and Shigematsu T: Environmental factors of cancer of the colon and rectum. Cancer 20:1520-1561, 1967.
28. Aries V, Crowther JS, Drasar BS, et al: Bacteria and the aetiology of cancer of the large bowel. Gut 10: 334-335, 1969.

THE ELUSIVE GONOCOCCUS

- **The control of gonorrhea in the United States is a critical challenge to the medical profession. A major effort will be required to meet this challenge.**

WINDER L. PORTER, M.D.

Twenty-five years ago, I attended a National VD Symposium where it was proclaimed that gonorrhea was on the run and we need no longer worry about it as we possessed the means to wipe the disease off the face of the earth. We are still suffering from the devastating influence of that false prediction. Though a few of us frantically cry out about the gravity of the situation, we just cannot generate the type of concern which needs to be addressed to this major public health problem. In the meantime, the gonococcus has developed new defenses and become progressively more elusive.

Just how serious is the problem? Last year in Delaware, the most frequently reported communicable disease was influenza. The second most frequent was gonorrhea with 1761 cases. This represented an increase from the previous year, when gonorrhea was number one, and continued a succession of years in which each reported annual incidence has exceeded that of the previous year. This annual increase in reported cases is seen throughout the United States where the increase has been over 14% in each of the last two years and 12% the year before that. The rise in infectious syphilis, the disease which forms the basis for most of our finanical support, appears to have been checked, at least nationally.

Whether the number of cases occurring each year is actually increasing to this extent can be questioned, for we know perfectly well that only a fraction of the cases are ever reported and it could be that a greater percentage of the cases have recently come to our attention. Also, it is frequent for patients to receive treatment without laboratory confirmation and without a report of any kind. We learn about these or see them only when failure, relapse, or reinfection ensues. The 1968 National Survey of Venereal Disease Incidence showed that four out of five cases of venereal disease were treated by physicians in private practice but that private physicians reported only about one out of every nine cases treated. From that survey it is estimated that nearly three-fourths of all the reported cases were those treated in public facilities and that more than one million other cases were treated by private physicians who made no report. Morever, there are many other cases which do not enter the statistics, either because gonorrhea is not suspected and not looked for, or because treatment is given without confirmation.

With so many hidden cases, distribution figures can be misleading for those who can afford the anonymity of private care are generally in better socio-economic circumstances and probably in a somewhat different age bracket. Of the cases reported in Delaware last year, 34% were between 20 and 24 years old, and another 28% were between 15 and 20. The age at which most cases are reported is 19 for males, and 18 for females. There is good evidence that the spread into higher age groups, particularly in the female, is greater than usually suspected and revealed only

Dr. Porter, M.P.H., is director, Bureau of Venereal Disease Control, Division of Physical Health, Department of Health & Social Services, State of Delaware.

when a concerted effort is made to detect and confirm infection in older patients.

The cardinal symptoms of gonorrhea in the male are urethral discharge and discomfort upon urination. A man who experiences these symptoms for the first time is apt to seek treatment, but it is entirely fallacious to believe that every infected male voluntarily seeks treatment. We regularly see patients who have been going around for three or four weeks with a supposed "strain" or "drip", and others who, when confronted with the opinion that they do have gonorrhea, offer sexual excitation or simple failure to wash as explanation for their symptoms. Some are carrying oral medication which they take according to their symptoms. Still others have no symptoms and are recognized only by culture or examination of the urinary sediment. This is particularly true of those who have been treated inadequately, especially with oral medication. And while a simple gram-stain is highly diagnostic in the acute state, a great many cases will be missed if dependence is placed upon smear alone especially in the less acute or those partially treated.

Epididymitis a Complication

A complication which now is being seen more frequently is epididymitis. Still fortunately uncommon are arthritis, septicemia, and endocarditis. Urethral stricture is much less common since we have abandoned meddlesome local medication and instrumentation, but acute involvement of the prostate is still encountered although less often leading to true abscess formation.

The gonococcus is notorious for starting a fight and then bailing out, leaving the field to other organisms, notably staphylococci and enteric pathogens which prolong the urethritis. While so-called NSU (non-specific urethritis) or NGU (non-gonococcal urethritis) may arise *de novo*, it is often an accompaniment or sequela of gonorrhea. Some of you may remember the early days of World War II when it was an offense punishable by court martial to contract venereal disease, and it was axiomatic that those above a certain rank did not contract gonorrhea, although it was acceptable for them to have NSU.

Incidence in the Female

Although women infected with gonorrhea may also have genital discharge and dysuria, many are truly asymptomatic. Vaginal discharge is such a frequent gynecologic complaint that it cannot be depended upon as a symptom unless of recent origin or altered in character. Besides discharge and urinary discomfort there may be pain and disturbances in menstruation, particularly what I call "stuttering menstruation" in which the patient reports that she thought she was having a regular period, wore a pad for a day or two, stopped, and then started bleeding again. When the Fallopian tubes are involved there may be severe abdominal pain, fever, anorexia, etc. — the familiar PID. While gonorrheal arthritis used to be seen more commonly in men, it now is more often seen in women, especially the pregnant, in whom it often presents as migratory polyarthritis easily mistaken for rheumatic fever.

The true incidence of gonorrhea in the female cannot be estimated for, as stated previously, it turns up much more often if suspected and looked for. There have been reports of incidence as high as 30% in correctional institutions, from 5 to 8% in prenatal clinics, from 5 to 30% in planned parenthood clinics and up to 8% in the offices of private physicians, not necessarily just those serving low income groups.

Culture is absolutely necessary to confirm the diagnosis, and specimens must be taken from multiple sites. The highest yield is obtained from the cervix, but it has been pointed out that the yield can be increased about 8% by including the rectum in addition to the conventional culture sites of the urethra and vagina. It was thought that special measures using an anoscope and taking pains to get the specimen from the crypts were needed to obtain proper rectal cultures but there is recent evidence of satisfactory results on specimens obtained from anal swab when care is taken to avoid feces. That a single negative determination is inconclusive is illustrated by one study in patients tested a week apart without treatment in the meantime. In this study, 6.4% were found positive on initial examination, but not at the repeat visit, and another 8.6% were turned up from among those who were negative on the first examination. In our situation we cannot await the results of confirmatory tests but must do what we can while we have our patients at hand; when in doubt, we treat.

I not infrequently am asked what to do with an infant whose mother has been found to have gonorrhea which was not known to be present at the time of her delivery. There can be no doubt that the time-honored Credé treatment has been highly efficacious in reducing the incidence of ophthalmia and that in the great majority of cases where gonorrhea is present and not suspected, the child gets by unscathed, so that in most instances it is safe merely to keep a close watch upon such an infant. Nonetheless where there is question about full cooperation in having the child followed, one may be justified in administering specific treatment. In some states, the physician is given the option of deciding what type of prophylaxis, if any, should be administered to infants' eyes. Almost always the highest percentage of failure is encountered when a procedure other than Credé has been employed, more often in the private or suburban hospital than in those which largely serve the inner city.

The risk to the infant is not confined to the eyes; infantile vulvovaginitis occurs more often after breech deliveries, and there have been sporadic reports of arthritis in the newborn and even of fatal septicemia. Not to be overlooked is the attendant at delivery; a physician I know lost an eye when membranes ruptured and there was a gush of gonococcal contaminated amniotic fluid into his face.

The treatment of choice for gonorrhea is still penicillin, and, as always, we have to say the proper dose is "enough." When the death knell of this disease as a public health problem was so freely predicted, our treatment consisted of 50,000 units repeated in three to four hours with entirely satisfactory results. Since then the recommended dose has slowly but steadily increased. When I re-

ported in the early fifties that we found it necessary to give much larger doses than usually recommended, I was pooh-poohed and told there was no such thing as penicillin-resistant GC and that other organisms were responsible, or these were reinfections.

Organisms Less Susceptible to Penicillin

As years passed, others came onto the bandwagon and it is now generally recognized that the gonococcal organisms are increasingly becoming less susceptible to penicillin. This situation is illustrated by the experience in Philadelphia where 52% of the organisms obtained by random culture in 1965 were susceptible to concentrations of penicillin less than 0.05 mcg/cc, while just three years later only 26% of the strains cultured were susceptible to the same concentrations. Perhaps the shift is more dramatically illustrated by another study where less than 3% of strains encountered in 1955 were resistant to concentrations below 0.5 units/ml while some 40% of strains cultured in 1965 were resistant to that concentration and more than 60% of those recovered in 1968-69 were resistant.

Now our regular initial dose is 2.4 million units of procaine penicillin for men and 4.8 million units for women. Even with these doses, some places are reporting as high as 30% failures and advocate that probenecid be added to prolong the action of the penicillin. It should be emphasized that cure requires a high blood level for a brief period, and delayed absorption preparations like benzathine penicillin may fail because of insufficient blood level.

We have made an effort to evaluate some other drugs in collaboration with Dr. Holloway. However, one must bear in mind that we do not have the type of close control possible in the military or in an institution. We may today see a patient who promises by all that is holy to return in two or three days so that we may evaluate response to treatment and yet we may not see him for two or three weeks, if at all. It is not safe to assume that those who fail to return have been cured, and it is never possible to be sure that reinfection is not responsible for what appears to be drug failure. Also in our situation, one cannot be satisfied with mere bacteriologic cure, for when the cultures are negative, the patient may still complain of discharge or of discomfort with urination. Penicillin has the advantage of effectiveness against a broad range of secondary organisms which account for persistent symptoms; ampicillin covers an even broader range but is too expensive for routine use. The tetracyclines also rank high in suppressing secondary organisms. What we are looking for is an alternative preparation which is relatively cheap, covers a wide spectrum, and can be administered in a single session. Oral medication is seldom taken as frequently or as long as it is prescribed. While many of the broad-spectrum antibiotics also are effective against syphilis, the doses given for gonorrhea would usually be quite inadequate to suppress concomitant infection with syphilis.

When I was invited to participate in this symposium, I felt that the subject of gonorrhea warranted enough consideration to consume the full time allotted. Since then there has been an epidemic increase in infectious syphilis. Instead of the average of about one new case per week that has been the pattern for the past several months, there has been a precipitous rise to 28 new cases in March, 21 of which were in the primary or secondary state. In assembling material for this presentation, I projected there would be 40 new cases for the month of April based upon the indicated trend. I overshot the mark by a couple of cases, but in these first few days of May the deficit has been made up.

These cases have turned up from all directions: from private physicians, from premarital and foodhandler examinations, from correctional institutions, from patients seen at each one of the local hospitals, and from epidemiologic investigation of other cases. An appalling realization is the number of these patients who had received attention elsewhere without recognition of the possibility of syphilis, having received salves for "hair cut" or "detergent" rash, oral medication for gonorrhea, and all kinds of pills, douches, and suppositories. One patient with florid lesions of secondary syphilis was told she had chicken pox.

At least ten of these patients had gonorrhea as well as syphilis, and some were seen initially because of that disease, including two or three who had lesions which they had not noticed or which they did not consider significant. Undoubtedly, others had gonorrhea which was not confirmed because treatment was initiated before definitive examination could be carried out. Another three have been treated for gonorrhea contracted since treatment for syphilis was completed. We make a practice of monitoring all patients treated for gonorrhea for the possibility of concomitant syphilis and can document for many the period within which they contracted syphilis on the basis of previous recent examinations. At this very moment, I am concerned about one who is in the seventh month of pregnancy and who had no satisfactory treatment because she claims to be allergic to penicillin and also has not been able to tolerate tetracycline.

The Resurgence of Syphilis

Part of the resurgence of infectious syphilis is attributable to cases which might have been curtailed or controlled by penicillin used to treat gonorrhea. It could well be that we will have to redirect our thinking and resume routine use of long-acting penicillin in addition to the high doses of short-acting penicillin recommended for treatment of gonorrhea.

For some time we have advocated that any female named as a sexual contact of a patient with gonorrhea should receive adequate treatment for gonorrhea even though she may not show any clinical or laboratory evidence of being infected. This policy has been extended to the homosexual male named as a contact and since this type of patient has been particularly involved in the current epidemic rise in syphilis, it is exceedingly important that particular attention be addressed to syphilis prophylaxis as a part of their management and that they be subjected to sustained surveillance.

So far most of the patients have been mature adults who have been married at one time, but the lower age range extends to 14 years. The chain of events has been entirely predictable as the stage was already set. It is not possible at this time to say that the tide has turned and that the spread has been checked even though now new cases are the subject of the most intensive epidemiologic investigation.

Just recently, I encountered a group of students from a nearby institution of higher learning who were staging what amounted to a mass "love-in" where they shared their affections indiscriminately with one another. One member contracted gonorrhea which he shared with his companions to the extent that except for one individual every member of the conclave was also proven to have contracted gonorrhea. They took it as a huge joke just as if it were scabies or body lice, which also are being seen more commonly. It could just as readily have been syphilis which they were bouncing back from one to the other and except for a mere happenstance, none of these kids might have come to our attention and received proper investigation. Or possibly, the first case might not have been recognized until the school year had terminated and others had dispersed in many directions.

With epidemic syphilis added to the tidal wave of gonorrhea patients for whom we lack sufficient facilities to handle properly, you can see we are in deep trouble. And as each patient emerges from our clinic, and tells his buddy the doctor's verdict, his friend mentally checks the links to see if he too is caught in the chain, and too often is forced to the conclusion, "I've got it too."

THE RAPID DIAGNOSIS OF GONORRHEA

• The lack of a rapid accurate method for the diagnosis of gonorrhea makes it necessary for the physician to treat all suspects or risk not treating active disease.

NANCY K. LARSON, B.A.
JANET L. CLARK, Ph.D.
WILLIAM J. HOLLOWAY, M.D.

In the diagnosis and treatment of gonorrhea, the clinician is faced with a dilemma—whether to treat all patients on the basis of a clinical suspicion of gonorrhea or to wait for laboratory confirmation and frequently lose infected patients for treatment and follow-up.

In the male patients, a gram-stain of the urethral discharge affords a quick means of diagnosis although a negative smear does not rule out the possibility of gonorrhea. In female patients, however, this method is not reliable at all and cultures are mandatory.

Cultural confirmation of the gonococcus by classical methods which use sugar fermentation for identification requires two to ten days, making the lapse between clinical suspicion and laboratory confirmation too long to delay treatment.

The usual fluorescent antibody (FA) method,[1] which consists of identifying organisms from growth on Thayer-Martin plates after incubation for 16-48 hours, has shortened the laboratory time and appears[2] to be as accurate as the culture method mentioned above.

This shortened laboratory time is more satisfactory than the classical culture method but still does not answer the clinician's need for immediate diagnosis. The direct fluorescent antibody technique, using a conjugate to stain the direct smears of urethral exudate, reduces the time to one hour, but also reduces the accuracy.[1,3]

This paper reports our evaluation of a more rapid (2.5 hours) fluorescent antibody method, attempting to provide a quick, reliable technique for detection of *N. gonorrhoeae*.

Material and Methods

Cultures were taken with cotton swabs which were immediately streaked onto Thayer-Martin plates. These plates were incubated for 16 to 48 hours and then suspected colonies were examined for *N. gonorrhoeae* by the FA method and confirmed by sugar fermentation. The same swab was then placed in 1.5 ml Mueller-Hinton broth to which had been added human serum (5%), IsoVitalex (Bio Quest) enrichment (1%) and V-C-N inhibitor (1%), the latter two being components of the Thayer-Martin medium. This tube was incubated in CO_2 at 35-37°C for two hours after which a smear was made from the swab. The broth was centrifuged at 2500 rpm for five minutes and the supernatant fluid decanted. The sediment was suspended in 1 ml PBS (pH 7.2), the tube centrifuged and the supernatant fluid decanted. A second smear was then made from the sediment. Both slides were air-dried, fixed and stained with the fluorescent conjugate which had been diluted with bovine albumin-rhodamine counterstain

Nancy Larson is Fluorescent Antibody Technologist, Dr. Clark is Coordinator of Research and Dr. Holloway is Director, Infectious Disease Research Laboratory, Wilmington Medical Center, Wilmington, Delaware.

79

(1:40). This stains the epithelial and white blood cells a red-orange color preventing the diplococci from being masked with non-specific fluorescence. Controls of *Staphylococcus aureus, Aerobacter cloacae, Mima polymorpha Oxidans* and other species of *Neisseria* were included to check the specificity of the staining.

Cervical and urethral cultures were obtained from 244 randomly selected patients at the Venereal Disease Clinic of the Wilmington Health Unit.

Results

N. gonorrhoeae was identified either by the rapid (two-hour incubation) FA method or by the delayed (24-hour incubation) FA method or by both methods in 83 (34%) of the cases. Positive cultures were obtained from 27 of the 114 females (23.7%) and from 56 of the 130 males (43.0%).

The patient population included those patients returning for posttreatment follow-up, so gonococcus was not anticipated in all patients from whom cultures were obtained.

Of the 244 specimens studied, there was agreement between the two methods in 234 (96%) cases. Positive identification by both the rapid and the delayed methods was made in 73 of 83 cases (88%). Five (6%) were positive by the delayed 24-hour method alone. Since it is possible that the few organisms present were left on the plate which was inoculated first, perhaps if two swabs had been used, one for the plate and one for the tube of broth, more of the broth cultures would have been positive. This is suggested because

the swab and the sediment were plated after the smears had been made, and in two cases no *N. gonorrhoeae* multiplication occurred. The other three cultures yielded organisms on subculture so the two-hour incubation was evidently insufficient in these cases.

Five specimens were positive after the short incubation but not the delayed method. It is most probable that these bacteria were not viable since plating the swab and the sediment produced no growth.

It would be desirable to have only one smear to evaluate, either from the swab which had incubated two hours in broth or the sedimented organisms from the broth. In over half (56.4%) of the cases, positive identification was made from both the swab and the sediment. If either of these methods had been used alone, however, 20-25% of the positives would have been missed. Calcium alginate swabs will be evaluated to determine if all of the organisms can be released into the broth, thus requiring only one smear, the sediment.

Based on these results, we have concluded that this method with a short (two hour) incubation method may have a place in venereal disease clinics equipped for fluorescent antibody procedures. Further trials seem warranted.

REFERENCES

1. Deacon WE, Peacock WL, Freeman EM, et al: Fluorescent antibody tests for detection of the gonococcus in women. Public Health Reports US 75:125-129, 1960.
2. Brown L, Copeloff MB and Peacock WL: Study of gonorrhea in treated and untreated asymptomatic women as determined by fluorescent antibody and culture methods. Am J Obstet Gynecol 84:753-757, 1962.
3. Price EV: Field evaluation of fluorescent antibody technique in the detection of the gonococcus in the female. Ann Symp Recent Advan Study Venereal Diseases (14th), Houston, Texas, 1964.

THE TREATMENT OF GONORRHEA WITH SPECTINOMYCIN AND RIFAMPICIN

• The prevalence of gonorrhea and the increasing incidence of treatment failure have prompted the study of new antibiotics in this disease.

RUSSELL LABOWITZ, M.D.
WINDER L. PORTER, M.D.
WILLIAM J. HOLLOWAY, M.D.

Recent periodic reports from the Public Health Service indicate that the incidence of gonorrhea is increasing in the United States. Several factors may be responsible for this increase: the short incubation period of the infection, the lack of immunity to repeated infections, and the increasing "resistance" of gonococcus to antibiotics, a particular problem with the Vietnam recruits.[1]

When penicillin was first available for the treatment of gonorrhea, N. gonorrhoeae was extremely sensitive to low concentrations of this antibiotic. However, in 1958, Curtis and Wilkinson[2] reported some strains of gonococci to be less sensitive to penicillin in vitro, and this observation correlated with a higher clinical relapse rate. Within the past decade, there has been reported an increase in the number of penicillin-insensitive strains which require higher serum levels of penicillin for eradication. The recommended dose of penicillin has been increased at regular intervals during the last few years in order to deal more effectively with this problem of increasing resistance. Despite this, there has been an increasing number of reports of treatment failures with supposedly adequate doses of penicillin. For example, the treatment of gonococcal urethritis in military personnel in the Far East with 2.4 million units of procaine penicillin results in 20-30% treatment failures. In a well controlled study[1] aboard an aircraft carrier, 63 men who recently had returned from leave in the Far East, were given 2.4 million units of procaine penicillin with 18 (29%) treatment failures.

It appears possible that future gonococcal strains will require even greater concentrations of penicillin, which would necessitate a therapeutic dose difficult to administer to an outpatient population. For this reason and because of the problem of penicillin allergy, new antigonococcal agents must be evaluated for their effectiveness in the treatment of gonorrhea. The ideal antigonococcal agent should be effective as a "one shot" treatment, easy to administer, non-toxic and not cross allergenic with penicillin.

In the last two years, we have had the opportunity to evaluate in the clinic two investigational antibiotics effective in vitro against Neisseria gonorrhoeae. Spectinomycin (Trobicin*) is an antibiotic produced by the fungus Streptomyces spectablis and has a wide spectrum of activity against both gram-positive and gram-negative organisms, including Neisseria gonorrhoeae. Rifampicin (Rifampin**) is a semi-synthetic antibiotic belonging to the group of rifamycins produced by Streptomyces mediterranei. It displays a high

Dr. Labowitz is a Fellow in Rheumatology, Arthritis Section, Hospital of the University of Pennsylvania Dr. Porter is Director of Venereal Disease Control. State of Delaware; and Dr. Holloway is Director of the Infectious Disease Research Laboratory, Wilmington Medical Center.

* Upjohn Company
** Dow Chemical Company

order of effectiveness *in vitro* against the gonococcus but most recently has received attention for its use in the treatment of tuberculosis.

Material and Methods

All patients were selected from the population of the venereal disease clinic. Most of the patients had had a previous history of gonorrhea and had received prior treatment with penicillin. All of the patients had clinical evidence of gonorrhea at the time of initial examination. Pre-and posttreatment urethral or cervical smears and cultures were done on each patient, and all positive cultures were confirmed by the fluorescent antibody technique. In addition, a routine urinalysis and VDRL were performed on each patient.

In the first study, female patients received 4.0 grams of spectinomycin intramuscularly (usually in two injection sites), while male patients received 2.0 grams intramuscularly. Follow-up visits were requested 48 hours and one week after treatment, at which time the patient was reexamined and recultured.

The second study was confined to male patients who received a single oral dose of 900 mg of rifampicin under the direct observation of the physician in attendance at the clinic. In addition to the cultures, urinalysis and VDRL, each patient treated with rifampicin had pre- and posttreatment blood counts and platelet estimations. Follow-up examination was requested 48 hours after therapy.

Results

A total of 85 patients was treated with intramuscular spectinomycin. Twenty-two patients were lost to follow-up. Eight patients were unsuitable for evaluation (five patients had negative pretreatment cultures, and three patients were classified as reinfections). Of the total of 55 patients that could be evaluated, 30 were male. In 26 of the male patients (87%), the results were satisfactory in that the patients were asymptomatic and posttreatment cultures were negative. Two patients (6.5%) were still complaining of dysuria and/or discharge after 48 hours although smears and cultures were negative and in two

patients (6.5%), there was bacteriologic failure.

Eighteen (72%) of the 25 females were treated successfully, while four female patients (16%) remained symptomatic despite negative smears and cultures. In three patients (12%), cultures remained positive. No significant side effects were noted except in one patient, who suffered transient dizziness 24 hours after the injection.

Rifampicin was used to treat 72 other cases of gonorrhea. Twenty patients were lost to follow-up, and reinfection could not be ruled out in two patients who returned to clinic beyond the two week follow-up period. Of the remaining 50 cases, 36 (72%) were treated successfully. Six patients (12%) were still symptomatic despite negative smears and cultures. Eight patients (16%) failed to respond (clinically and bacteriologically) even though the pretreatment strains were sensitive to rifampicin. In two of these eight patients, the posttreatment organisms were completely resistant to rifampicin by disc and a third had only a 10 mm zone. This raises the question of development of resistance *in vivo*. It is interesting that four patients who were treated successfully with rifampicin became reinfected and received a second course of rifampicin therapy. The pretreatment strains in all four patients were sensitive to rifampicin. The second treatment was successful in two patients and failed in one patient. In the fourth patient the culture was negative, but the patient still had symptoms, including urethral discharge.

Neutropenia and cholestatic jaundice have been reported to be associated with rifampicin treatment, usually in patients on maintenance therapy, but no hematological abnormalities or jaundice was noted in this study. One patient did complain of transient diarrhea within 24 hours after taking the drug.

Discussion

It appears from this limited study that intramuscular spectinomycin is an adequate treatment for acute gonorrhea in male and female patients. On the other hand, experience with rifampicin in 50 male patients with gonococcal urethritis suggests that this agent is not as promising in the treatment of gonorrhea. The apparent development of resistant strains in four patients following therapy casts doubt on the potential value of rifampicin as an alternative drug for the treatment of gonorrhea.

No serious side effects were noted from either antibiotic. One patient complained of transient dizziness following spectinomycin therapy.

Sixteen percent of the females treated with spectinomycin were still symptomatic despite negative cultures. This is disconcerting because in the absence of satisfactory, rapid diagnostic tests, retreatment of symptomatic patients is mandatory. Frequently the persistence of clinical evidence of disease is due to pathogens other than the gonococcus. A number of these female patients had abundant trichomonads, identified on smears, which may have contributed to their symptomatology. In a recent report by Tsao,[3] 620 patients (42%) of 1,466 patients with culturally proven gonorrhea had concomitant trichomoniasis.

There may be one or more causes for the so-called post-gonococcal urethritis (PGU). Whether this entity represents persistence of gonorrhea (perhaps in the L-form stage), a concomitantly acquired non-gonococcal urethritis such as trichomoniasis, T-strain myco-plasma infection, or just a slow resolution of urethral inflammation following adequate therapy, has yet to be determined. In any event, the occurrence of PGU is increasing even after "adequate penicillin" therapy. In a prospective study[4] done on a ship, PGU was present in nearly two-thirds of 58 men treated with procaine penicillin and probenecid.

Summary

Because of the relatively small size of this study, no categorical statements can be made about the clinical efficacy of these two drugs. Continued clinical trials are necessary to find the ideal antigonococcal agent. In the meantime, the resistance patterns of the gonococci in this country must be followed very closely and the search for alternative treatments continued. At the present time, "penicillin resistant" gonorrhea is more of a problem in military personnel in Southeast Asia than in the United States. However, with the recent return of thousands of troops from Vietnam, the problem undoubtedly will become greater in this country.

REFERENCES

1. Holmes KK, Johnson DW and Floyd TM: Studies of venereal disease. I. Probenecid-procaine penicillin G combination and tetracycline hydrochloride in the treatment of "penicillin-resistant" gonococcus in men. JAMA 202:461-466, 1967.
2. Curtis FR and Wilkinson AE: A comparison of the in vitro sensitivity of gonococci to penicillin with the results of treatment. Brit Journ of Venereal Disease 34:70-78, 1968.
3. Tsao W: Trichomoniasis and gonorrhea. Brit Med Journ 1:642-643, 1969.
4. Holmes KK, Johnson DW, Floyd TM, et al: Studies of venereal disease. II. Observations on the incidence, etiology and treatment of the post gonococcal urethritis syndrome. JAMA 202:467-473, 1967.

CEPHALEXIN IN THE TREATMENT OF GONORRHEA

• Cephalexin, an oral cephalosporin, produces blood levels comparable to those resulting from parenteral cephalosporin administration. Therefore, evaluation of the efficacy of this new antibiotic in gonorrhea is indicated.

WILLIAM A. TAYLOR, M.D.
WILLIAM J. HOLLOWAY, M.D.

Over the last several years, gonorrhea has become an increasingly important and difficult public health problem. Complicating factors are the increase in the number of cases of gonorrhea (494,945 reported in 1969 with an estimated 1,000,000 unreported cases[1]) and the increasing *in vitro* resistance of strains of *Neisseria gonorrhoeae*.[2] An additional problem is the occurrence of penicillin allergy in patients requiring therapy for gonorrhea. These problems have prompted the investigation of new antibiotics in the treatment of gonorrheal infections.

Before the reported efficacy of newer antibiotics such as the cephalosporins and kanamycin (Bristol), one used tetracycline or erythromycin (Eli Lilly) to treat resistant or recurrent cases of *Neisseria gonorrhoeae* infection. The success of Lucas and co-workers[3] in treating gonorrhea in male patients with a single intramuscular dose of two grams of cephaloridine (Eli Lilly), prompted the evaluation of the effectiveness of cephalexin (Eli Lilly), a new orally administered cephalosporin, in males with acute gonococcal urethritis.

Cephalexin monohydrate is the first oral cephalosporin antibiotic to produce high serum levels.[5] Clinical experience has shown this antibiotic to be effective in the treatment of soft tissue and urinary tract infections.[6-8] Since orally administered cephalexin gives serum levels comparable to those resulting from an

intramuscular dose of cephaloridine,[9] it was reasonable to expect that this antibiotic might be effective in the treatment of gonorrhea.

Material and Methods

Thirty male patients with clinical evidence of gonococcal urethritis were selected for treatment with cephalexin monohydrate. The antibiotic was administered in a single oral dose of three grams, the total dose being swallowed under the supervision of the clinic physician. Before treatment, urethral cultures were obtained and the swabs streaked on Thayer-Martin agar. Bacteriologic confirmation was obtained by identification of colonies characteristic of *Neisseria gonorrhoeae* by oxidase testing and subsequently by fluorescent antibody staining techniques. Blood specimens were obtained from all patients included in the study for VDRL determination. Patients were asked to return 48 hours after administration of this antibiotic for clinical and bacteriologic follow-up. At this time, patients were interviewed to determine the existence of side effects from the antibiotic.

The strains of *Neisseria gonorrhoeae* obtained from patients in this study were tested for sensitivity to cephalexin by the disc-agar diffusion technique and by the test-tube dilution technique employing Mueller-Hinton broth.

As a corollary to this study, blood and urine levels of cephalexin were determined in 12 volunteers following the administration of three grams of cephalexin by mouth in fasting

Dr. Holloway is Director, Infectious Disease Research Laboratory, Wilmington Medical Center, Wilmington, Delaware and Dr. Taylor is Resident-in-Medicine, Wilmington Medical Center.

and feasting states. Serum levels were drawn at one-half, one, two, four, six and 12 hours after administration of the three-gram dose of antibiotic. In addition, all volunteers had complete blood counts, SMA-12 chemistry profile, and urinalysis carried out before and after administration of the three-gram dose of cephalexin. The serum levels for cephalexin were performed in the Eli Lilly Laboratory for Clinical Research, utilizing a cup plate microbiological assay with *Sarcina lutea* as the test organism.

Results

Ten of the 30 patients treated with cephalexin failed to return for follow-up examination. Twelve of the 20 patients who did return for follow-up were clinical and bacteriologic cures, while six of the patients were judged as failures by both clinical and bacteriologic parameters. Two additional patients were apparent bacteriologic cures but continued to complain of mild dysuria associated with a discharge. The clinical failures were subsequently treated with either 2.4 million units of procaine penicillin or twelve grams of tetracycline divided over a three-day period. There were no side effects noted during the study, and there were no positive tests for syphilis in the 30 patients from whom blood was drawn.

Cephalexin Serum Concentration

Serum levels following the ingestion of three grams of cephalexin in a fasting state in 12 volunteers were as follows: one-half hour 56.1 mcg/ml, one hour 77.6 mcg/ml, two hours 58.4 mcg/ml, four hours 14.5 mcg/ml, six hours 3.4 mcg/ml, 12 hours 0.3 mcg/ml. When the same volunteers were given three grams of cephalexin one hour following a meal, the serum levels were as follows: one-half hour 20.9 mcg/ml, one hour 59.9 mcg/ml, two hours 88.1 mcg/ml, four hours 27.8 mcg/ml, six hours 8.1 mcg/ml, and 12 hours 0.7 mcg/ml. These results suggest that administration of cephalexin in a feasting state delayed the peak level of cephalexin in the serum but did not lower the height of the final peak. These results disagree somewhat with those obtained by other investigators[10] who found that the peaks were lower and later. There were no

side effects noted in the volunteer studies nor were there any changes noted in the pre- and posttreatment toxicity studies.

Sensitivity Studies

Seventeen strains of *Neisseria gonorrhoeae* obtained during the clinical trial survived subculture to undergo sensitivity testing. All of these strains were inhibited in the test tube by 0.4 to 3.1 mcg/ml of cephalexin. Disc sensitivities utilizing a 30 mcg disc showed zones of inhibition of 15-30 mm. Follow-up cultures obtained from the bacteriologic failures did not show evidence of increasing resistance to cephalexin.

Comment

Cephalexin, a new oral cephalosporin antibiotic, has been shown to be clinically effective in the treatment of urinary tract and soft tissue infections. It is readily absorbed from the gastrointestinal tract producing excellent blood and urine concentrations, and clinical experience to date has shown a low order of toxicity. The desirability of obtaining more oral agents effective in the treatment of gonorrhea when given in a single dose prompted the study of this agent in the treatment of acute gonococcal urethritis in male patients. A 30% failure rate was obtained in this limited study suggesting that a single three-gram dose of cephalexin is not a satisfactory alternative treatment for acute gonococcal urethritis. At the present time, studies are underway at our clinic to evaluate the use of a three-gram dose of cephalexin enhanced by a one-gram dose of probenecid in the treatment of male patients with acute gonococcal urethritis.

REFERENCES

1. Schroeter AL and Pazin GL: Gonorrhea. Annals of Inter Med 72:553-559, 1970.
2. Martin JE, Lester A, Price EV, et al: Comparative study of gonococcal susceptibility to penicillin in metropolitan areas of the United States. Ninth InterScience Conference on Antimicrobial Agents and Chemotherapy, 1969. In Press.
3. Lucas JB, Thayer JD, Utley PM, et al: Treatment of gonorrhea in males with cephaloridine. JAMA 195:919-921, 1966.
4. Keys TF, Halverson CW and Clarke EJ: Single dose treatment of gonorrhea with selected antibiotic agents. JAMA 210:857-861, 1969.
5. Wick WE: Cephalexin, a new orally absorbed cephalosporin antibiotic. Applied Microbiology 15:765-768, 1967.
6. Page J, Levinson ME, Thornhill TS, et al: Treatment of soft tissue infections with cephalexin. JAMA 211:1837-1839, 1970.
7. Levinson ME, Johnson WD, Thornhill TS, et al: Clinical and in vitro evaluation of cephalexin: A new orally administered cephalosporin antibiotic. JAMA 209:1331-1336, 1969.
8. Hogan LB: Cephalexin in the treatment of urinary tract infections. Seventh Annual Infectious Disease Symposium, 1970. Del Med Journ. In Press.
9. Perkins RL, Carlisle NH and Saslaw S: Cephalexin: in vitro bacterial susceptibility, absorption in volunteers and antibacterial activity of sera and urine. Amer Journ of Med Science 256:122-129, 1968.
10. Griffith RS and Black HR: Cephalexin: A new antibiotic. Clin Med 75:14-22, 1968.

8th
INFECTIOUS
DISEASE
SYMPOSIUM

ANTIBIOTIC COMBINATIONS

- Expertise in the use of antimicrobial agents requires familiarity with the advantages and disadvantages of the administration of antibiotics in combination.

MAXWELL FINLAND, M.D.

There has been a great deal written in recent months about drug combinations, the great bulk of it in the so-called "throwaways" — the "controlled circulation" journals and medical newspapers which are operated for profits they derive largely, or almost exclusively, from pharmaceutical advertising. It is also a lively subject of discussion in trade journals, and, from time to time, even in the general news media — usually on their financial pages. Some of this material has been contributed by respected academic and practicing physicians who have taken issue with certain of the recent evaluations made by the panels of experts who re-evaluated the efficacy of drugs approved by the US Food and Drug Administration (FDA) between 1938 and 1962. These evaluations were conducted under the aegis of the National Academy of Sciences-National Research Council (NAS-NRC) and with guidelines which the FDA has now proposed to adopt for the approval of all new drugs in fixed combinations.

I shall not dwell on the history of the drug laws, beginning with the Pure Food and Drug Act of 1906, which was designed primarily to prevent adulteration of foods and drugs, and later the Food, Drug and Cosmetics Act of 1938, which required proof of safety of all new drugs, and culminating in the Drug Amendments of 1962 (also referred to as the Kefauver-Harris Amendments), which require proof of efficacy as well as safety of all new drugs before they can be approved for prescription by physicians. The background of these laws and the various amendments and regulations are well summarized and ably presented in Dr. Harry F. Dowling's carefully prepared, scholarly, well balanced and very readable book, recently published under the title *Medicines for Man.*[1]

The various panels of experts, using guidelines prepared after consultation and with the general approval of representatives of industry, the FDA, the Policy Advisory Committee of the Drug Research Board (DRB) of the NRC and all the panel chairmen, considered the many claims of the manufacturers for the efficacy of each of the drug combinations they were marketing. They concluded, from all the data and literature available to them, and based on their own expert opinions, that there was insufficient evidence to warrant these claims for the great majority of drug combinations available in fixed dose ratios, which they were asked to review. This was particularly true of the five panels of 30 experts who dealt with anti-infective drugs; these particular panels were further guided by a special policy statement on fixed combinations of antimicrobial agents which was prepared by two of the panels and adopted by the members of the other three panels.[2] Some of the conclusions and recommendations of the Panels on Anti-Infective Drugs dealing with fixed combinations have already been implemented without objections by the manufacturers; others were put into effect after "hearings" or after litigation in the courts; and the others, for a variety of reasons, are still under review by the FDA.

During the heated discussions that have been going on in the press, in the medical literature and at various meetings, there have been many confusing and contradictory statements about drug combinations. In particular, the subject of fixed combinations has been confused with that of multiple drug therapy; and the combinations of pharmacologic agents

Dr. Finland is Epidemiologist, Boston City Hospital; George Richards Minot Professor of Medicine, *Emeritus,* Harvard University, Boston, Mass.

have been equated with those of antimicrobial agents in fixed-dose ratios. Examples have often been cited of multiple drug therapy, or even some drugs available in fixed ratios, which are accepted as well proved but which are not necessarily among those rated by the panels as ineffective.

When Dr. Holloway invited me to participate in this Symposium, I thought this might offer an opportunity to review the subject as related to my own area of competence, namely, antibacterial drugs. For this purpose, I propose to present, in a more or less didactic fashion, without detailed documentation, but with some brief comments, the facts I have been able to gather from the literature, relating to the general subject of multiple drug therapy and particularly to fixed combinations of antibacterial agents.

Major Reasons for Prescribing Combinations of Antibacterial Agents

The following are some of the justifications for prescribing more than one antibacterial agent and the problems they raise, or factors which must be considered when they are used:

1. *To broaden the therapeutic range so as to include organisms not adequately affected by one of the agents when used alone*

When used for this purpose the choice of drugs should be based on a definite or highly probable bacteriological diagnosis and the known effectiveness of the drugs selected against the probable causative organisms.

2. *For life-threatening infections until a definite bacteriological diagnosis is established*

Under such circumstances one may select either a) the most suitable single agent that is most effective against the most likely causative organism, or b) multiple specific agents, each against a different, but likely, causative bacterial agent. A single, broad-spectrum drug is often, but not always, preferable to multiple agents. In any event, it is essential to obtain materials from all sources — blood, urine, sputum and exudate — for culture *before* starting treatment, so that the appropriate therapy, generally with the single most effective agent, may be used and others discontinued as soon as the correct etiologic diagnosis is established.

3. *To prevent, delay or reduce the degree of resistance that may emerge before bacteriological cure is effected*

This indication arises particularly in the treatment of tuberculosis, chronic pyelonephritis, endocarditis or other deep-seated or inaccessible infections in which a) the causative organism is known to acquire resistance rapidly (resistant mutants emerge), or b) the antibiotic is known to induce resistance rapidly. Examples of such organisms are: *Staphylococcus aureus*, *Mycobacterium tuberculosis*, and some strains of *Proteus* and of *Escherichia coli*. Examples of such drugs are streptomycin, erythromycin, novobiocin, rifampin and nalidixic acid. If used for these indications, each agent must be active against the causative organism by a different mechanism or at a different site; it should have similar pharmacokinetics, but there should be no cross-resistance between or among the agents used.

4. *To suppress or prevent overgrowth of other bacteria that are already present, or which might be acquired*

This may be justified if directed against a single, highly susceptible organism, eg, penicillin and group A hemolytic streptococcus, sulfadiazine and a susceptible meningococcus, or an active antistaphylococcal agent against a known susceptible strain during an influenza epidemic associated with a high prevalence of severe staphylococcal pneumonias. It has been invoked by using a penicillinase-inhibiting penicillin as a means of suppressing penicillinase production by staphylococci to permit the action of penicillin G. These uses are of limited values because a) the anti-penicillinase activity has not been regularly achieved *in vivo*, b) it is not possible to suppress all pathogens, and c) resistant ones tend to emerge to colonize or to cause superinfections.

5. *To suppress fungi and yeasts during therapy with large doses of broad-spectrum or multiple antibacterial agents*

Such use does not prevent overgrowth or superinfection by other organisms, such as *Proteus* or *Staphylococcus*.

6. *To reduce the dose-related toxicity by using smaller amounts of each agent*

Such a mechanism can be invoked for closely related drugs. However, each agent may contribute its own peculiar type of toxic effect.

7. *To utilize different pharmacokinetics*

Agents with different properties of diffusion into cells, cerebrospinal fluid, bile, or serous cavities are used for this purpose. Examples are given in subsequent sections.

Some Useful Combinations of Similar Antimicrobials

There are a number of examples of such combinations which have been used to a varying extent.

1. *Two or three sulfonamides*

The combination of sulfapyrimidines (sulfadiazine and its methylated derivatives—sulfamerazine and sulfamethazine) has been recommended and used effectively in equal amounts of each. When so used, they have an additive effect, with reduction in the occurrence of crystalluria because each has its individual solubility which is unaffected by the presence of the other, thus reducing the crystalluria, hematuria, and renal tubular obstruction resulting from the full dose of the single component. The indications are the same as for the individual components or other sulfonamides, primarily for urinary tract infections.

2. *Streptomycin and dihydrostreptomycin*

The eighth nerve toxicity of the former is primarily vestibular, and that of the latter is primarily cochlear, but each may produce both effects, and the use of equal parts of each was considered as possibly reducing both types of toxicity. This combination was exploited for a while in the treatment of tuberculosis but has generally been abandoned because the cochlear effect was not really prevented. Moreover, dihydrostreptomycin is no longer recommended for systemic use in this country.

3. *Procaine penicillin with aqueous penicillin G and benzathine penicillin*

Combination of two or all three of these three forms of penicillin has been recommended as initial therapy or for use as a single dose to take advantage of the different rates of absorption of each of these forms. The indications are the same for penicillin G,

mainly for the treatment of gonorrhoea or for the treatment or prevention of group A hemolytic streptococcal infections.

4. *An isoxazolyl penicillin plus penicillin G*

This combination has been recommended and used to secure the action of penicillin G and to broaden its spectrum so as to include some resistant staphylococci and gram-negative bacilli, but its clinical effectiveness is not established.

Combinations of Dissimilar Antimicrobials Reported as Being Useful

1. *Penicillin plus streptomycin*

For several years this combination was the one most frequently employed, particularly by surgeons, for its supposed broad spectrum, or to initiate therapy, or for prophylaxis in mixed infections. In the fixed combination it was used extensively where penicillin alone was indicated. In appropriate dosage of each it has been shown to be synergistic *in vitro* and *in vivo* against many strains of *Streptococcus faecalis* and has been used successfully in the treatment of endocarditis due to this organism. Much ototoxicity, including deafness, has resulted from the prolonged, unnecessary, and irrational use of this fixed combination.

2. *Various combinations of dissimilar agents active against the same causative organisms*

The best example is the use of two or three dissimilar antimycobacterial agents for tuberculosis (isoniazid, with paraminosalicylic acid and streptomycin or with ethionamide or ethambutol). The multiple therapy, each in full doses, is given to prevent or delay the emergence of resistant tubercle bacilli. Combinations of active antistaphylococcal agents are also used in the treatment of endocarditis or osteomyelitis, when one of the agents has a high mutation rate, such as erythromycin or streptomycin. These are rarely called for now that effective cephalosporins and penicillinase-resistant penicillins are available.

3. *Penicillin plus sulfonamides*

This combination is offered for its broad spectrum and for the different pharmacokinetics and modes of action of the components. It has been used in the treatment of meningitis, actinomycosis and other susceptible infections.

4. *Chloramphenicol plus streptomycin or a sulfonamide*

These drugs given together presumably offer favorable pharmacokinetics in the management of meningitis due to gram-negative bacilli.

5. *Tetracycline plus amphotericin B or nystatin*

The antifungal agent is given when oral tetracycline is indicated in young children and in women with the purpose of suppressing yeasts and fungi and preventing thrush and vaginitis due to *Candida*. Although this seems quite rational, it has been difficult to find adequate, consistently significant clinical confirmation.

Antibiotic Combinations Shown to Be Synergistic in Vitro

Synergy has been variously defined, but it generally refers to an action or rate of antibacterial action of two agents together which cannot be achieved by either one separately, or which requires significantly smaller amounts of each to achieve the same or greater biological effect. Such action has been demonstrated by many workers with various combinations against selected species and strains of pathogens. Some of the most prominent and some recent examples may be cited.

1. *Penicillin plus either streptomycin, kanamycin or gentamicin or with vancomycin*

Such combinations, as already noted, have been used with success in the treatment of enterococcal endocarditis. Synergy has been demonstrated against selected strains of *Proteus mirabilis* and *P. vulgaris*.

2. *Ampicillin or cephalothin plus streptomycin or kanamycin*

These combinations have exhibited synergy against some strains of *Klebsiella, Enterobacter, E. coli* and *Proteus*.

3. *Carbenicillin plus gentamicin or polymyxin*

Evidence for synergy of these combinations against some strains of *Pseudomonas aerugi-*

nosa has been shown to be strain specific. More recently carbenicillin plus gentamicin have been shown to exhibit antagonism *in vivo* with apparent reduction in the activity of the gentamicin during concomitant administration of carbenicillin in some cases, although clinical evidence of a favorable synergistic effect has been reported by several workers in a number of cases of pseudomonas infections.

4. *Ampicillin or penicillin G plus either cloxacillin or nafcillin or cephalothin*

These combinations of a penicillinase-sensitive penicillin with a penicillinase inhibitor have been shown to act synergistically against selected strains of *Pseudomonas, Enterobacter* and *Proteus morganii* (but not against strains of other species of *Proteus*). Some cases of urinary tract infections due to strains of *Pseudomonas* which have exhibited such synergy *in vitro* have apparently responded to treatment with the same combination.

5. *Tetracycline plus oleandomycin*

The synergy against resistant *S. aureus* on which the introduction of this combination was based and justified has not been confirmed.

6. *Penicillin G plus erythromycin*

Some evidence for synergy of this combination against strains of *S. aureus* that were resistant to each agent separately has been presented, this has indeed been confirmed by several workers, but antagonism of this combination against some susceptible strains has also been encountered. To my knowledge this has not been marketed as a fixed combination in the United States.

7. *Penicillin plus either tetracycline or chloramphenicol*

Various species of enterobacteria, including some of *Salmonella*, have shown synergy to these combinations.

8. *Polymyxin B plus sulfadiazine (1:20)*

Only strains of *Serratia marcescens* are affected synergistically by this combination in this ratio.

9. *Polymyxin plus chloramphenicol*

Some strains of *Pseudomonas* are acted on by this pair of antibiotics synergistically.

10. *Tetracyclines plus either streptomycin or penicillin*

Synergy with the streptomycin combination against *Brucella* has been demonstrated *in vitro* and in clinical studies, but clinical reports confirming the *in vitro* synergy of tetracycline with penicillin in the treatment of brucellosis are not available to confirm this action.

11. *Ampicillin plus chloramphenicol*

Synergy of this combination has been reported against strains of *Salmonella*, but adequate proof of such an action in patients with salmonellosis is not available.

12. *Trimethoprim plus sulfamethoxazole (1:5)*

This combination is clearly synergistic in this ratio against many bacterial strains and species. Both components act by a similar mechanism at different stages of the synthesis of folate. Although the optimal ratio for synergy may vary for different species or strains *in vitro*, the 1:5 ratio is the one that has been reported as being effective in a number of clinical trials in Great Britain and in other countries. It is now under clinical trial but not yet available in this country.

Antibiotic Combinations Reported as Showing Antagonism

The antithesis of synergy, ie, reduction in the antibacterial effect or rate of killing by one agent when used in combination with another, is called antagonism. Such an effect is less common than synergy but has been clearly demonstrated with some combinations of antimicrobials against some species, or individual strains. The following are among those that have been reported *in vitro*.

1. *Penicillin plus a tetracycline or chloramphenicol*

Both of these combinations have been found to exhibit antagonism *in vitro* against *Streptococcus*, *Pneumococcus* and *Klebsiella pneumoniae*, and in infection of mice with some strains of these organisms. Antagonism of penicillin and chlortetracycline has been demonstrated in experimental pneumococcal infections in mice, and also clinically in the treatment of pneumococcal meningitis and in scarlet fever.

2. *Penicillin G plus erythromycin*

As already noted, this combination, which may show synergy against *S. aureus*, has exhibited an antagonistic effect against some strains of group A hemolytic streptococcus and also in the treatment of cases of scarlet fever due to this organism.

3. *Penicillin G or kanamycin plus chloramphenicol*

These combinations have been found to be much less active than either agent alone against a number of strains of *Proteus mirabilis*.

4. *Ampicillin plus polymyxin B or colistin*

Antagonistic effects of these combinations have been reported against some strains of *Salmonella*.

5. *Streptomycin or kanamycin or nalidixic acid plus either chloramphenicol or tetracycline*

Each of these combinations has shown antagonism against strains of *Proteus*.

6. *Erythromycin or other macrolides plus lincomycin or clindamycin*

These combinations of agents, which act at the same cytoplasmic site on the same ribosomes, are completely antagonistic *in vitro* against strains of *S. aureus* and other susceptible species. There is no evidence of such antagonism *in vivo*.

7. *Penicillin G plus streptomycin*

Antagonistic action of this combination against some strains of *Pseudomonas* has been reported.

8. *Ampicillin plus chloramphenicol*

This combination, which may act synergistically against some strains of *Salmonella*, has been reported as showing definite antagonism against *Hemophilus influenzae in vitro*. This is an important observation, which has not been recognized in the treatment of meningitis due to this organism, but should be kept in mind as a possible explanation for relapses in patients treated with these agents, which are commonly employed for that purpose in young children.

Some Incompatibilities of Antibiotics

Many failures of antibiotic therapy are associated with improper use of the antibiotics. A number of such failures have been traced to incompatibilities of these agents when mixed together or when administered in certain menstrua.

1. *The following antibiotics have been found incompatible when mixed with others for intravenous injection:*

Amphotericin B
Cephalosporins (cephalothin, cephaloridine)
Chloramphenicol
Colistimethate
Erythromycin (or other macrolides such as oleandomycin)
Lincomycin or clindamycin
Novobiocin
Polymyxin B
Rifampin
Tetracyclines (all analogues)

2. *The following have been found to be incompatible with antibiotics for parenteral therapy and should not be mixed with them:*

Calcium gluconate or chloride
Corticosteroids
Heparin (this may be used before and after the antibiotic is injected but not together)
Pressor amines (with potassium salts)
Vitamins, single or multiple

3. *Oral neomycin plus penicillin G or V or phenethicillin*

The absorption of each of these oral penicillins is reduced when given with oral neomycin.

Undesirable Aspects of Uncritical Use of Antimicrobial Combinations Particularly Those Available in Fixed Ration

1. It is not possible to make any absolute generalization concerning the usefulness or undesirability of any combination against any microbial species or strains; successful results have been rare, whereas false expectations are frequent and disappointing.

2. Multiple antimicrobials may produce hy-

persensitivity and other untoward reactions to more than one of the drugs, including those that are not contributing any useful antibacterial activity (eg, to novobiocin or triacetyloleandomycin when given together with tetracycline; ototoxicity from streptomycin when combined with penicillin).

3. Resistance to one or both components of the combination may be present or develop and render the combination ineffective, as when streptomycin is given with penicillin, or when novobiocin or oleandomycin is given with tetracycline.

4. The drugs may suppress but not eradicate the causative organism and delay or make it difficult or impossible to establish a bacteriological diagnosis.

5. The possibility of colonization and superinfection is increased when multiple antibiotics are used, and the new organisms or infections are then resistant to all of the antibiotics that were used.

6. The fixed combinations generally provide inadequate dosage for serious infections that respond to only one of the agents if given in full doses.

7. It is rarely possible to include a proper fixed dose ratio of any two or more antimicrobials that will provide adequate treatment for infections for which they are intended. One possible exception: trimethoprim and sulfamethoxazole, a combination currently under investigation.

8. The physician is confused by poorly documented, testimonial types of endorsements and by deceptive or misleading advertisements of combinations as though they are new and more active drugs when more often they contain agents which the physicians have already used without success.

9. There is an unnecessary increase in cost when the combinations are used, particularly when single ones are adequate.

REFERENCES

1. Dowling HF: Medicines for Man: The Development, Regulation and Use of Prescription Drugs. New York, A A Knopf, 1971
2. Drug Efficacy Study. Final Report to the Commissioner of Food and Drugs, Food and Drug Administration, from the Division of Medical Sciences, National Research Council — National Academy of Sciences, Washington, DC, US Gov Printing Office 1969.

COMPLICATIONS OF ANTIMICROBIAL THERAPY

• All of the antimicrobial agents available for use in man are capable of producing significant side effects. The practicing physician must select the proper antibiotic in the treatment of an infectious disease, and he must also be aware of the possible side effects of the agent that he selects.

MARVIN TURCK, M.D.

Although antimicrobial agents have had a generally favorable impact on many human infections, they have often been a double-edged sword by exerting their toxic effects on both the microbe and the host. At times the complications of treatment are inevitable and predictable and clearly are related to interference with essential metabolic function of normal cells. At other times undesirable effects seem to be specific for a given host, are idiosyncratic and largely unpredictable. Finally, in some instances the side effects of these drugs are due to their ability to upset the delicate biologic balance between microorganism and host, resulting in bacterial resistance and superinfection.

There have been numerous excellent reviews[1-5] of the dangers inherent in antimicrobial therapy, and only the more important developments will be summarized. The discussion will deal with six different categories of drugs:

1. The penicillins and cephalosporins
2. The broad-spectrum agents
3. Agents effective primarily against gram-positive bacteria
4. Agents effective primarily against gram-negative bacteria
5. Antifungal antibiotics
6. Sulfonamides and other agents useful in infections of the urinary tract

Penicillins and Cephalosporins

The penicillins and cephalosporins presently

Dr. Turck is Associate Professor of Medicine, University of Washington, and Chief of Medicine, United States Public Health Service Hospital, Seattle.

in clinical use are relatively nontoxic for mammalian tissue. However, there is some evidence that the semisynthetic penicillins may have inherent toxicity not found in the parent compound, benzylpenicillin. For example, a few cases of neutropenia, renal functional impairment, and elevations of serum glutamic oxaloacetic transaminase have been reported following administration of methicillin, oxacillin or carbenicillin. It should be remembered also that all of the penicillins are capable of causing central nervous system excitation and convulsions when administered in very high doses, especially to patients with pre-existing renal disease. In addition, experience with the antimicrobial cephaloridine has suggested that this agent may be potentially nephrotoxic and should be avoided in patients with underlying renal disease. The main advantage of cephaloridine over cephalothin is that parenteral injection is better tolerated. Occasionally treatment with cephalothin and other cephalosporin antibiotics has resulted in the appearance during therapy of a positive Coombs test. This has not been associated, however, with a hemolytic anemia as, for example, is the case with alphamethyldopa.

Most of the untoward reactions to this group of antibiotics are not toxic but are related to hypersensitivity, and are usually characterized by urticaria or other erythematous skin eruptions. Less frequently the penicillins and the cephalosporins cause fever and arthralgias resembling serum sickness. There is probably complete cross-allergenicity among the true penicillins, and it seems prudent to avoid, in patients with a history of a penicillin reaction, rechallenge with any of this group of drugs including the semisynthetic congeners. Ampicillin appears to have a lower incidence of immediate anaphylactoid reactions than does penicillin G. This difference may be due to traces of a proteinaceous constituent of the fermentation brew detectable in penicillin G, and even in 6-aminopenicillanic acid, but not in the semisynthetic penicillin derivatives. Delayed reactions, on the other hand, occur more frequently with ampicillin. In a recent report of drug surveillance among almost 4000 patients, rashes occurred in 9.5% of patients treated with ampicillin, 4.5% of those treated with other penicillins, and 1.8% of individuals not given these drugs. Furthermore, eruptions beginning after the first week of treatment were much more common with ampicillin. Another peculiarity of ampicillin is its tendency to cause a morbilliform, macular-papular eruption rather than urticaria. In addition, there is a propensity for patients with infectious mononucleosis to develop rash following treatment with ampicillin. Whether or not these are "true" penicillin reactions is not presently known.

Although the similarity between the cephalosporin nucleus (7-amino-cephalosporanic acid) and penicillin nucleus (6-amino-penicillanic acid) suggests that cross allergenicity may be a problem, degradation of cephalothin, cephaloridine, cephaloglycin and cephalexin proceeds along different pathways from those followed by penicillin. Nevertheless, extreme caution in administering a cephalosporin to a patient with known previous penicillin hypersensitivity reaction is indicated since there have been patients in whom an identical reaction has followed administration of both penicillins and cephalosporins.

There is some evidence that superinfections may be more frequent among patients treated with the newer penicillins or cephalosporins than in those given penicillin G. This may be related to the higher dosage of the new agents and also to the use of these drugs in more severely ill and debilitated patients whose skin and mucous membranes may already be colonized with gram-negative organisms prior to treatment with antimicrobials.

Broad-Spectrum Agents

Although several antibiotics may be effective against common gram-positive and gram-negative pathogens, mycoplasma, and rickettsia, the term broad spectrum generally has been associated with the tetracycline group of antibiotics and with chloramphenicol. The term will be used in this context.

Both toxic and hypersensitivity reactions are uncommon when tetracyclines (tetracycline hydrochloride, oxytetracycline, chlortetracycline, demethylchlortetracycline, methacycline and doxycycline) are used in recommended dosage, and most undesirable effects consist of gastrointestinal disturbances. Fungal (*Candida*) overgrowth leading to glossitis, stomatitis, pruritus ani and vulvae is more common with the tetracycline group of antibiotics but is more bothersome than hazardous. Most of the serious side effects are related to suppression of the normal bacterial flora, resulting in superinfection, particularly with resistant *Staphylococcus aureus*. Staphylococcal enterocolitis and pneumonia may be insidious in onset and may be fatal.

More recently there has been noted a group of heretofore less recognized complications. One of these, photosensitivity, is more frequent with demethylchlortetracycline, and patients receiving this drug should avoid sunlight. The tetracyclines have also been shown to have antianabolic activity resulting in nitrogen retention in certain susceptible patients, particularly those with pre-existing azotemia and renal failure. These drugs have also been incriminated in causing acute hepatic necrosis, followed by renal failure, especially in pregnant or post partum women to whom tetracyclines were administered in relatively large doses by parenteral route. An unusual complication has been the occurrence of a Fanconi-like syndrome related to the use of outdated oral tetracyclines. This has been attributed to degradation products of the drugs and, fortunately, has been reversible. Finally, when infants and children were exposed to these drugs early in life or *in utero*, mottling and discoloration of the teeth and abnormal deposition of the drug in bones have been reported.

Chloramphenicol continues to be a well-tolerated antibiotic and causes few hypersensitivity type reactions. In newborns, especially prematures, treated with more than 50 mg/kg/day it may cause the gray syndrome, which is characterized by lethargy, cyanosis, and a peculiar pallor. The syndrome, which has been attributed to an accumulation of chloramphenicol in the blood stream related to immaturity of the glucuronyl-transferase system in the newborn, may culminate in circulatory collapse and death.

More pertinent to the problem, is the relatively rare but extremely important hematotoxic potential of chloramphenicol. There are at least four things which may happen to the blood-forming apparatus of patients given chloramphenicol: 1. Slight transient leukopenia may occur; this is usually of little consequence. 2. One may see large, vacuolated, normoblastic cells in the bone marrow. Whether this stage of chloramphenicol toxicity is a fore-runner of aplastic anemia is not clear. These cells are also seen in other disturbances of erythropoiesis and may not be specific for chloramphenicol toxicity. 3. An interesting observation has been the deleterious effect of chloramphenicol in anemic patients. For example, it has been shown that patients with iron deficiency anemia fail to respond to iron with reticulocytosis as long as they are receiving chloramphenicol, and it is not until the drug is withdrawn that blood values return to normal. Similar observations have been made with vitamin B_{12} in pernicious anemia. 4. Complete necrosis of the bone marrow with consequent aplastic anemia, agranulocytosis and, more rarely, thrombocytopenia may occur.

There are a number of clues which should lead the clinician to suspect that chloramphenicol is interfering with erythropoiesis. A high serum iron, high saturation of iron-binding protein, and absence of reticulocytosis have all been helpful in detecting chloramphenicol toxicity. Unfortunately, however, there is no iron-clad guarantee that these abnormalities herald the early onset of marrow aplasia. In fact, many workers feel that there is little relation between these abnormalities and the subsequent development of bone marrow failure. Although the mechanism for the marrow aplasia is unknown, it is felt by some that the interaction of chloramphenicol with certain gut bacteria may lead to a toxic degradation product. Pertinent to this point, there seems to be no recorded case in which marrow aplasia has followed administration of chloramphenicol by parenteral routes alone. This, however, may merely be a chance observation related to the inordinately greater number of patients given chloramphenicol by mouth. In either case, the best rule of thumb in employment of chloramphenicol is to use this drug only in severe infections in hospitalized patients in whom sensitivity tests or the clinical picture dictates that chloramphenicol is superior to other available drugs. Never should this drug be administered prophylactically and rarely for prolonged periods.

Agents Active against Gram-Positive Bacteria

This is a group of antibiotics whose primary usefulness lies in the realm of gram-positive infections in patients with penicillin allergy.

Erythromycin and oleandomycin are macrolide antibiotics similar in antibacterial activity. Toxic and hypersensitivity reactions are uncommon; superinfections are also rare. Gastrointestinal discomfort is the main untoward effect and is more common with high dosages. Loose stool and diarrhea with these drugs probably are associated with an increase in gastrointestinal motility rather than to a change in bowel flora. Hepatotoxicity, manifested primarily by an elevation in bilirubin and alkaline phosphatase, has been associated with a modified preparation of erythromycin (the lauryl ester of erythromycin propionyl sulfate) and of oleandomycin (triacetyloleandomycin). Although these dosage forms are associated with increased antibacterial activity, perhaps related to better absorption, jaundice will develop in some patients. Presumably, this toxic effect is a consequence of competition for conjugating enzymes. The icterus disappears promptly upon discontinuing the drugs, and permanent hepatotoxicity probably does not occur.

Lincomycin and 7-chloro-lincomycin (clindamycin) are closely related antibiotics effective against many common gram-positive pathogens, including most staphylococci. These drugs are nontoxic and relatively non-allergenic, and lincomycin, at least, is well tolerated by both oral and parenteral routes. Gastrointestinal discomfort is the main drawback. Clindamycin is associated with increased antibacterial activity in serum, perhaps related to better absorption.

Vancomycin is a potent antistaphylococcal and antienterococcal antibiotic and is most useful in seriously ill patients who are allergic to penicillin. Its main drawback is that it must be administered intravenously and is frequently associated with thrombophlebitis and pain. Nephrotoxicity has been reported in a very small percentage of patients; some investigators attribute this to impurities in some of the original preparations of vancomycin. The major untoward effect of vancomycin is ototoxicity resulting in permanent deafness. This complication has been observed primarily in azotemic individuals with impaired renal function. A small number of patients have also developed a hypersensitivity type reaction to vancomycin manifested by chills, fever, rash and vascular collapse. Pretreatment with antihistamines may prevent this side effect.

Novobiocin enjoyed temporary vogue in the treatment of staphylococcal infections before the availability of the semisynthetic penicillins and was marketed primarily in the form of a novobiocin-tetracycline combination. Several untoward reactions ranging from mild gastrointestinal disorders and skin eruptions to fever and severe jaundice have been reported with this drug. A metabolic breakdown product of this glycoside antibiotic causes yellow discoloration of the skin and mucous membranes independent of its effect on the liver.

Bacitracin should be administered only by the topical route. It is bactericidal against the common gram-positive organisms and is virtually without side effects when used topically. Although the drug is nonallergenic and resistance to it is seldom found, parenteral administration is painful and is associated regularly with impaired renal function culminating in both glomerular and tubular damage. Since the advent of safer antistaphylococcal antibiotics, parenteral administration of bacitracin is rarely, if ever, justified.

Agents Active against Gram-Negative Bacteria

There are a number of antibiotics including streptomycin, kanamycin, gentamicin, neomycin, colistin (polymyxin E) and polymyxin B, with an antibacterial spectrum directed primarily against gram-negative pathogens.

Streptomycin, kanamycin, gentamicin and neomycin have similar chemical, pharmacologic and toxic properties. Neomycin is probably the most toxic of the group, but the others are also associated with significant toxicity primarily to the auditory nerve and the kidney. The ototoxic effects of streptomycin and probably of gentamicin are associated with destruction of the vestibular nuclei and with lesions of the terminal fibers of the eighth cranial nerve. Kanamycin and neomycin affect the auditory portion of the nerve. Although deafness and vestibular malfunction have usually followed excessive, repeated or prolonged administration of one of these drugs, permanent damage has also occurred with ordinary doses administered for as short a period as seven days. These complications have been more frequent in elderly patients, especially those with pre-existing renal disease.

Nephrotoxicity with streptomycin, characterized by casts, red cells and proteinuria in the absence of previous renal disease, is seldom observed nowadays because highly purified preparations of streptomycin are the only ones used. Nephrotoxicity associated with neomycin and kanamycin is related both to dose and total duration of treatment. With neomycin nephrotoxic effects are uncommon if therapy does not exceed 1.0 gm/day for seven days. In patients with pre-existing renal disease this dosage must be decreased, and blood levels should be monitored. These same principles apply to kanamycin, and a total course of therapy should not exceed 20 gm in adult patients with normal renal function. Although less is known about the nephrotoxic potential of gentamicin, there is every reason to suspect that it has a similar propensity to cause nephrotoxicity. Interestingly enough, these drugs appear relatively less toxic in infants than in adults.

Ordinarily, absorption from the gastrointestinal tract is negligible with streptomycin, kanamycin, neomycin and gentamicin; however, when these drugs are administered orally to patients with ulcerative disease of the bowel or decompensating liver disease, absorption may increase and toxic levels can be reached, particularly if there is concomitant renal failure.

An unusual untoward effect of these agents has been the production of respiratory arrest following their intraperitoneal or systemic administration at the time of surgery; this is especially prone to occur in patients concomitantly receiving curare-like neuromuscular inhibitory drugs. There have been also instances of a myasthenia gravis-like syndrome reported with these drugs.

Although not common, these agents are capable of evoking hypersensitivity type reactions with fever and eosinophilia. Contact dermatitis has occasionally followed prolonged exposure to neomycin and streptomycin. Finally, when these drugs are given orally some patients develop a severe watery diarrhea, which may progress to a sprue-like illness even after diarrhea has subsided. In other instances, fulminant staphylococcal enterocolitis has developed during oral treatment with neomycin. Patients with decompensating hepatic disease who are receiving this drug to abort or reverse hepatic coma are particularly susceptible to this complication.

Colistin and polymyxin B have similar antibacterial activity and toxicity when expressed in therapeutically equivalent doses. Their toxicity, which is dosage dependent, is exerted mainly on the nervous system and kidney. Renal disturbances are usually completely reversible and consist of transient azotemia and changes in the urinary sediment. Neurologic symptoms are related to the ability of the polymyxins to inhibit neuromuscular transmission and vary from mild paresthesia, especially around the mouth, to severe vertigo, ataxia and, at times, complete paralysis. These symptoms usually subside within seventy-two hours of discontinuing treatment and do not leave lasting residua. The polymyxins are decidedly more toxic in patients with pre-existing renal disease, in whom blood levels and kidney function should be carefully monitored. True allergic reactions are uncommon. One apparent advantage of colistin over polymyxin B is less pain at the site of intramuscular injection, which may be related solely to the addition of the local anesthetic, dibucaine, to colistin.

Antifungal Antibiotics

Currently there are three effective antifungal antibiotics in general clinical use. Nystatin and griseofulvin are useful for surface infections, and amphotericin B for systemic infections.

Nystatin and griseofulvin are largely nontoxic when administered by mouth. Nystatin is poorly absorbed, and its main usefulness is for the topical treatment of muco-cutaneous monilia infections. It has also been used prophylactically along with broad-spectrum antibiotics in an attempt to suppress fungal superinfection. Griseofulvin is absorbed from the gastrointestinal tract and is effective in controlling many superficial fungal infections of the skin, hair and nails. Amphotericin B is the primary drug available for treatment of systemic mycotic infections. It must be administered by intravenous route (or intrathecally in some cases of meningitis) and causes a variety of side effects. The most frequent side reactions consisting of chills, fever, nausea, vomiting and headache, are marked during the first treatment periods and diminish in intensity as treatment progresses. Phlebitis is also common following intravenous administration. These undesired effects may be minimized by premedication with aspirin or an antihistamine and addition of a small amount of hydrocortisone to the infusate.

The three major toxic effects associated with amphotericin B are anemia, which occasionally is severe enough to require transfusions, hypokalemia, which may necessitate potassium supplementation, and nephrotoxicity. Continued use of the drug has been associated with irreversible kidney damage and a peculiar, intrarenal calcification. Usually, however, azotemia and functional impairment are reversible, although recovery after amphotericin B is discontinued may be protracted, and in some instances the renal lesions never heal completely.

Sulfonamides and Other Urinary Tract Antimicrobials

The sulfonamides remain the drugs of choice in the initial treatment of urinary tract infections in patients with no history of recurrent urinary infections or of urinary tract obstruction. Although they have been used for a number of years and are relatively safe, they have the potential for causing untoward reactions. There is some evidence that the long-acting preparations may carry a greater risk of reactions than the other sulfonamides. In concentrated urine, sulfonamides can crystallize in the tubules; fortunately this occurs infrequently with the newer, acetylated compounds. The sulfonamides can also lead to hemolytic anemia in patients with a deficiency of glucose-6-phosphatase in red blood cells. Other unusual reactions include skin rashes, hemolytic and aplastic anemia and other bone marrow disturbances, renal and hepatic toxicity, myocarditis, drug fever, and arthritis. Sulfonamides also have been associated with defects in bilirubin metabolism, especially in premature infants, and have been implicated in kernicterus. Fortunately, most of these toxic, allergic and idiosyncratic reactions are mild or uncommon.

Nitrofurantoin is another antibacterial agent used primarily in the treatment of patients with infection of the urinary tract. The main untoward reactions are epigastric distress, nausea, and vomiting which can be minimized by taking the drug with meals. There is some evidence that a new macromolecule of nitrofurantoin, Macrodantin, is better tolerated. Similarly to the sulfonamides, nitrofurantoin may cause hemolysis in patients with glucose-6-phosphatase deficiency. It has also been associated with a pleural-pneumonia syndrome, eosinophilia, and rash and has been found to cause peripheral polyneuritis, especially in elderly patients with renal impairment, a few of whom have died or have been left with permanent neurologic deficits.

Nalidixic acid also has various reactions, which, in general, have been reversible. These have included gastrointestinal upset, urticaria, pruritus, rash, convulsions, transient visual disturbances, and photosensitivity. The excretion products may give a false positive test for glucose in the urine when tested with reagents such as Benedict's solution, a consequence of the liberation of glucuronic acid from nalidixic glucuronide.

REFERENCES

1. Dunlop DM and Murdock JM: The dangers of antibiotic treatment. Brit Med Bull 16:67-72, 1960.

2. Gale EF: The nature of the selective toxicity of antibiotics. Brit Med Bull 16:11-15 1960.

3. Feingold DS: Antimicrobial chemotherapeutic agents: The nature of their action and selective toxicity. NEJM 269:900-907, 957-964, 1963.

4. Weinstein L: Chemotherapy of microbial diseases. The Pharmacological Basis of Therapeutics. Goodman L and Gilman A ed. Section XIV, pp 1144-1307, New York, MacMillan Co, 1965.

5. Smith TJ: Antibiotic-induced diseases. Diseases of Medical Progress. Moser RH ed, pp 3-60, Springfield, Charles C Thomas, 1964.

ANTIMICROBIAL SUSCEPTIBILITY TESTING —

Its Value and Limitations in Medical Practice

• Carefully performed laboratory susceptibility tests can provide assistance to the physician in his selection of antimicrobial agents. However, the clinician and the laboratory technician must be aware of the limitations of these laboratory procedures.

ALLAN R. RONALD, M.D.

During the past decade, the proliferation of antimicrobics has made the problem of selecting the best therapy for the individual infected patient inordinately complex. In order to make this decision correctly the physician must know the susceptibilities of the infecting organisms; he must understand the disease process, its natural history and the possible influence of antimicrobic therapy; he must be informed about the toxicity absorption, distribution, and excretion of the antimicrobics available for therapy. This paper will concern itself with the first point, ie, the susceptibility testing in the laboratory. This is now a major part of the workload of the diagnostic laboratory.

First, we must define the terms sensitive and resistant. The following criteria are suggested:

1) The organism is sensitive if it is inhibited by considerably less (by a factor of 2 to 4 fold) than the average blood levels attained with an ordinary dose. Conversely, resistance implies that the organism would not be effectively inhibited by blood levels attained with an ordinary dose. This does not take into account special situations such as the urinary tract where antimicrobials may be concentrated many fold.
2) A bimodal distribution of susceptibility often emerges as organisms within a species develop resistance to an antimicrobic.

Strains that fall in the less susceptible population are considered resistant.
3) Clinical studies demonstrate a correlation between the response to therapy and the *in vitro* prediction of susceptibility.

These definitions do not take into account special host factors such as drug absorption and excretion, the drug level at the site of infection, or the role played by the host in controlling and eradicating the infection. In addition to the categories of sensitive and resistant, some laboratories provide an intermediate category. This implies that if the organism is present in the urine it may be eradicated by the urinary level of the antimicrobic.

As well as providing essential information for patient care, the laboratory obtains an additional bonus from sensitivity testing. Antibiograms have become important taxonomic tools that are used every day in pigeon-holing organisms. For example, how often do tetracycline-sensitive *Proteus mirabilis* occur? Also, these same criteria can play a major role as biologic markers in studying the epidemiology of hospital infection and may be more readily available than phage typing for labelling common hospital pathogens such as *Staphylococci*.

This paper will not go into methodologic details. However, regardless of the techniques a few general principles apply to all techniques and bear repetition. First, studies can only be done on pure cultures. It is grossly

Dr. Ronald is Assistant Professor, Departments of Medical Microbiology and Medicine, University of Manitoba and the Winnipeg General Hospital, Winnipeg, Manitoba, Canada.

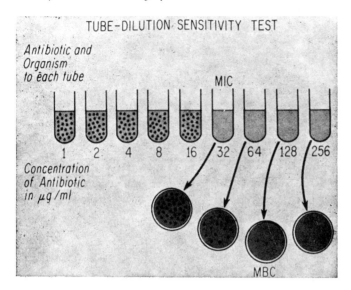

Figure 1

Pictorial depiction of the tube dilution susceptibility test.

misleading to report sensitivities based on discs placed directly on streaked specimens except in instances in which a pure culture of the pathogen can be anticipated. Second, for routine sensitivity testing to be reproducible in any laboratory, careful quality control is required. This must include the media and the antimicrobics as well as the conditions of the test method. Third, a well standardized, widely adopted procedure should be used for routine work. Any changes in the media, inocula or other methodologic detail will alter the interpretative criteria of the method and must be carefully evaluated before being placed in routine use. Unfortunately, the lack of standardization of sensitivity methods has resulted in great variations in results from laboratory to laboratory. This problem will be solved only if physicians and microbiologists insist that sensitivity procedures be widely standardized and uniform across the country.

Methods for In Vitro Sensitivity Testing

Three commonly used methods for *in vitro* sensitivity testing are available.

The broth dilution technique is depicted in Figure 1. The dilutions of antibiotic are prepared to cover a meaningful clinical range. A standard inoculum of organism is added to each tube. After incubation, usually over-

night, the lowest concentration of antibiotic that inhibits the organism is called the minimum inhibitory concentration or MIC. Subcultures from the tubes that initially appear clear, that is showing inhibition, are made to determine the minimum bactericidal concentration or MBC. Automation of the broth dilution in a microtiter system has been developed in several laboratories and may make this a more routine test.

Figure 2 depicts the agar dilution method. Antibiotics, in this case ampicillin, are diluted in solid media so that each plate represents one concentration. The MIC is read at the lowest concentration which prevents growth.

Both these dilution methods are useful, and one of them should be available in every microbiology laboratory. They do provide a number which is intended to relate to the level of antimicrobic in the patient. Unfortunately, these methods can give varying results depending on the conditions of the test situation. Also, it is impossible to reproduce in the test tube the *in vivo* conditions that may obtain in a particular lesion.

Most laboratories depend for routine sensitivity testing on the agar disc diffusion meth-

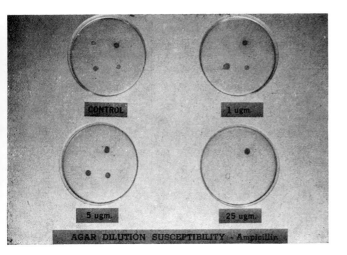

AGAR DILUTION SUSCEPTIBILITY - Ampicillin

Figure 2

Agar dilution susceptibility with four organisms with varying resistance to ampicillin.

od. This test is convenient, and readily performed, and well standardized methods are available. An agar plate is seeded with the organism and discs placed firmly on the agar. The antibiotic in the disc diffuses into the surrounding agar, inhibiting the growth of the organism. This results in the zones of inhibition around the disc. The size of the zone depends on a great many factors including the amount of antibiotic in the disc, the diffusibility of the drug, the susceptibility of the organism, and its rate of growth. This is shown in Figure 3.

Figure 4 depicts the relationship between the zone of inhibition plotted on the abscissa and the $\log_{10}$ of the MIC plotted on the ordinate. For any given drug, there is an approximate linear relationship between these two values. That is, the disc diffusion test performed in a standardized manner provides quantitative information, and an estimation of the MIC of the organism can be made. However, the diameter of the zone of inhibition around one antimicrobic cannot be compared with the size of the zone of inhibition of other antimicrobics. Each drug must be standardized for itself. Also, the amount of antimicrobic in the disc does not in any way relate to the MIC of the organism. For example, a zone around a 10 unit penicillin disc does not imply that the organism is susceptible to 10 units.

Guidelines for Selection of Organisms

General guidelines for selection of organisms for antimicrobial sensitivities include the following:

1) Organisms thought to be responsible for specific infection should be tested. Sensitivity tests should not be done on organisms that are a part of the normal flora and are not acting as pathogens in the clinical setting. In some laboratories, personnel may have considerable responsibility in deciding the organisms to be tested for antimicrobial sensitivity. Results reported on normal flora may lead to useless and even dangerous treatment by suggesting that these organisms have an etiologic role in the infection.

2) Routine sensitivities are not required on organisms with predictable sensitivity patterns. This includes pneumococci, group A streptococci, gonococci, and meningococci. However, even here survey studies should be done every few years to ascertain that this pattern has not changed. Also, whenever an infection presumed to be due to a uniformly sensitive organism fails to respond to that antibiotic, sensitivity tests are indicated. During the past few years, these methods have detected the emergence of resistant organisms on a number of occasions. For example, patients

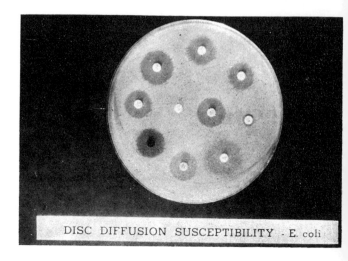

Figure 3

Agar diffusion susceptibility test
on 150 mm. Petri plate using the
Kirby-Bauer technique.

DISC DIFFUSION SUSCEPTIBILITY - E. coli

with pneumococcal pneumonia failing to respond to tetracycline have been discovered in retrospect to have infection with tetracycline resistant *D. pneumoniae*. Surveys have subsequently defined that about 10% of group A streptococci and 3% of pneumococci are resistant to tetracycline. The discovery of sulphonamide resistant meningococci and penicillin resistant gonococci followed a similar pattern.

3) Organisms that develop resistance rapidly on exposure to antibiotics should be tested prior to therapy and again if isolated during therapy. Some antimicrobics permit rapid emergence of resistance. For example, in about 20% of patients treated with nalidixic acid, the pretherapy sensitive organism becomes resistant.

Selection of Antibiotics

The spectrum of antimicrobics to be routinely tested will vary from area to area and should be developed jointly between the clinicians treating patients and the laboratory director. The following antimicrobics are used routinely in the Winnipeg General Hospital.

Staphylococcus aureus: Sensitivities should be routinely performed whenever it is considered to be a pathogen. The following antimicrobics should be routinely tested:

	% resistant
— penicillin (ampicillin not necessary)	60
— a penicillinase resistant penicillin (oxacillin)	rare
— cephalothin	rare
— erythromycin	10
— lincomycin	2
— tetracycline	15
— kanamycin	3
— vancomycin	100

Staphylococcus epidermidis: This organism is occasionally a pathogen. It is a problem in sepsis from intravenous catheters. The same antimicrobics as for *S. aureus* should be tested. Oxacillin (methicillin) resistance is much more common and occurs in 5 to 10%.

Non-group A streptococci (includes enterococci): These organisms require routine sensitivities if thought to be a pathogen. Recent tests of enterococcus reveal that 70% are resistant to penicillin and cephalothin, 20 to 30% are resistant to erythromycin, tetracycline, and nitrofurantoin and rare strains are resistant to ampicillin.

Clostridium species: Routine sensitivity testing is unnecessary as they are predictably sensitive to the penicillins, cephalosporins, erythromycin, and tetracyclines and resistant to the aminoglycoside antimicrobials.

Gram negative species other than Pseudo-

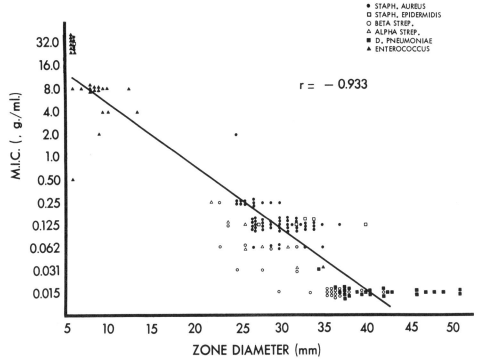

Figure 4 — Comparison of antibiotic discs and agar dilution tests of susceptibility with clindamycin.

monas: These organisms should be tested with ampicillin, cephalothin, tetracycline, chloramphenicol, kanamycin, and gentamicin. Nitrofurantoin, nalidixic acid, and sulphonamide should be included only if the organism is from the urinary tract.

Pseudomonas aeruginosa: This organism is predictably resistant to cephalosporins, ampicillins and nalidixic acid. It should be tested against tetracycline, chloramphenicol, gentamicin, carbenicillin, sulphonamide, and polymyxin or colistin.

Miscellaneous Organisms

a. *Neisseria meningitidis* are predictably sensitive to penicillin. However, sulphonamides remain the only effective antimicrobial for eradicating the carrier state. At present, at least 50% of meningococci are sulphonamide resistant. Bennett[1] has shown that sul-

phonamide sensitivity determined with a disc technique on Mueller-Hinton agar can accurately predict sensitive organisms and correlate with the agar dilution technique.

b. *Neisseria gonorrhoeae* have gradually become more resistant to penicillin. Sensitivity tests preferably by the agar dilution method are indicated in patients who have failed to respond to penicillin.[2] Fortunately, with a dose of 2-4 million units of penicillin, a cure is still effected in over 90% of the patients. At present, the tetracyclines are the alternate drug of first choice.

c. *Listeria monocytogenes:* These organisms are predictably sensitive to ampicillin and tetracycline.

d. *Hemophilus influenzae:* These organisms are predictably sensitive to ampicillin, chloramphenicol and tetracycline, and routine sensitivity tests are not indicated. Surveys should be done periodically.

e. *Anaerobic gram-negative rods (Bacteroides)* have been predictably sensitive to chloramphenicol. Most strains originating in the mouth are sensitive to penicillin or ampicillin. Tetracycline has been a most useful drug, but at present resistance to this antimicrobic is not unusual. Lincomycin and more recently clindamycin and vancomycin have been used successfully to treat patients with these infections. Unfortunately sensitivity tests with these organisms are difficult and have not been well standardized. The diffusion tests can be used with organisms that grow well enough within 24 hours to determine zones of inhibition.

The physician is under constant pressure to use newer antimicrobics. The laboratory is also often coerced into using the discs of these newer agents so that the physician will be presented with the sensitivities for the wonderful new agent "Marvelomycin." The decision as to what antimicrobics should be tested in the laboratory should be made by both the clinicians and the microbiologist. The antimicrobics chosen should have been shown to be effective in reputable clinical studies, and *in vitro* criteria for sensitivity testing should have been well worked out. The laboratory shares the responsibility with the physician if patients are treated inadequately because improper antimicrobics are selected.

Of the ordinary penicillins, only penicillin G need be tested. Only one of the semisynthetic penicillinase-resistant penicillins should be tested. Oxacillin is more stable than methicillin, and with the disc method oxacillin has been shown to better predict staphylococcal resistance to the penicillinase resistant penicillins.[3] Carbenicillin sensitivities should be performed for *Pseudomonas*. This new semisynthetic penicillin has increased the antibacterial breadth of the penicillin family by including many strains of *Pseudomonas*, the indole positive *Proteus*, and some *Enterobacter* in its spectrum. Criteria for interpreting disc sensitivities still remain to be established and for the present, dilution sensitivities are being used.

Cephalothin discs can be used for all the cephalosporins. Erythromycin and lincomycin are both useful agents in coccal infections and merit sensitivity testing.

Only one of the tetracyclines, preferably tetracycline itself, should be tested. There is no logical reason for reporting sensitivities to doxycycline, methacycline and demethylchlortetracycline. To do so only confuses the physician and wastes laboratory time.

Chloramphenicol sensitivities should be restricted to the gram-negative organisms and its use discouraged except in specific indications such as typhoid fever.

The aminoglycoside antibiotics, kanamycin and gentamicin, have become very important therapeutic agents in the treatment of gram-negative infections. Streptococci and all anaerobics are predictively resistant, and when they are used in the treatment of very ill patients with undiagnosed infection, this must be kept in mind. When gentamicin was first introduced, resistant *Enterobacteriaceae* or *Pseudomonas* were essentially non-existent. At present, in the Winnipeg General Hospital where gentamicin has been widely used for four years, gentamicin-resistant *Enterobacteri*-aceae are rare, but about 5% of *Pseudomonas* are resistant. The emergence of organisms resistant to this antibiotic needs to be carefully monitored in order to forestall the emergence of widespread gentamicin resistance.[4]

Sulphonamide sensitivity testing continues to be criticized despite several excellent studies showing clinical correlation with *in vitro* sensitivity. Media free of sulphonamide inhibitors (eg, Mueller-Hinton agar) should be used and the same criteria applied as in other sensitivity testing.[5]

Nitrofurantoin and nalidixic acid sensitivities should be performed on gram-negative organisms isolated from urine. The sensitivity tests with these drugs are based on urinary drug levels.

Methenamine mandelate is a clinically useful agent in the prevention of recurrent urinary infection but has a more limited role in the treatment of infection. As it is only active at an acid pH, sensitivity studies are of no value and should not be done.

Occasionally, the laboratory is requested to perform sensitivity tests with combinations of two or more antimicrobials. Fortunately, these are not used as frequently as in the past and at present should only be done in special situations such as enterococcal endocarditis. Various combinations of penicillin and streptomycin or ampicillin and streptomycin should be tested using a tube dilution technique with subcultures to give bactericidal end-points.

In conclusion, we need to be continually reminded that the laboratory's task is not complete until the physician caring for the patient has the results of the work. This frequently requires personal communication in order that delays in effective therapy do not occur.

REFERENCES

1. Bennett JV: Rapid sulfonamide disc sensitivity test for meningococci. Applied Micro 16:1056, 1968.
2. Ronald AR, Eby J and Sherris JC: The susceptibility of *Neisseria gonorrhoeae* to penicillin and tetracycline. Antimicrobial Agents and Chemotherapy, 1968. Amer Soc Microbiology, Ann Arbor, Mich p 431-434, 1969.
3. Drew WL, O'Toole R and Sherris JC: Failure of cloxacillin discs to detect resistance of *Staphylococcus aureus* to penicillinase resistant penicillins. Abstract in the Ninth Interscience Conference on Antimicrobial Agents and Chemotherapy, p 71, 1969.
4. Snelling EFT, Ronald AR, Cates C, et al: Studies of gram negative resistance to gentamicin. J. Infect Dis (In Press)
5. Bauer AW and Sherris JC: The determination of sulfonamide susceptibility of bacteria. Chemotherapia (Basel) 9:1, 1964.

PREVENTION AND TREATMENT OF
RESPIRATORY VIRAL INFECTIONS IN CHILDREN

● The outbreaks of viral respiratory infections in Australia closely resemble those that occur in the United States. Influenza vaccine and amantadine have been shown to be effective in preventing influenza.

STANLEY W. WILLIAMS, M.D.

As a pediatrician, one has the impression that in most respiratory infections of childhood, the cause is not known and defies detection by the most modern laboratory techniques. A "cold" can be due to one of four prevailing viral infections in our community — parainfluenza, adenovirus, respiratory syncytial virus (R.S.V.), or Coxsackie B. A streptococcal infection of the throat can cause similar symptoms. The trigger mechanism for most cases of bronchial asthma is also unknown, and could be related to viral infection.

Although the known respiratory viruses tend to cause typical syndromes, Stuart-Harris[1] states none is specific for a particular clinical syndrome. Chanock[2] and more recently Gardner[3] have defined the roles of parainfluenza viruses in the causation of croup and bronchiolitis. The significance of the isolation of a virus in the course of an illness concerns us as to whether the virus is a pathogen. Gardner[3] states that parainfluenza and R.S.V. are seldom isolated except when the patient has symptoms. There are many viral respiratory diseases for which we have no cure or prevention, and on the other hand, there seem to be potential chemotherapeutic agents for which there is, so far, no appropriate disease.

Some epidemics and sporadic endemic respiratory viral infections are reasonably clarified, even if unpredictable, and this applies particularly to influenza viral infection. With the approach of winter in Australia, considerable thought is being given to the necessary steps to cope adequately with the likelihood of viral epidemics, especially influenza.

Prediction

Except in 1957, when the epidemic of A_2 Asian influenza in Australia preceded that in the United States, our epidemics follow the pattern of those in the United States and Europe. As influenza A_2/Hong Kong has been present in Australia each year from late 1968 to 1970, it is unlikely this will recur in 1971. As you know, influenza B has occurred recently in the United States[4] with the absenteeism from some schools reaching 20 to 30 per cent, indicating sporadic epidemics, and possibly that is what will happen in Australia. Of considerable interest has been the incidence of 36 cases of hepatoencephalopathy (Reye's syndrome).

There were a few isolations of influenza B in Melbourne towards the end of winter in 1970, and this virus could be endemically dormant in our community — or it will flare up by contacts from outside the country. Australia last had an influenza B epidemic in 1965, so that children under the age of six years will be susceptible and could possibly benefit by immunization.

Dr. Williams is Consultant Pediatrician, Royal Children's Hospital, and Consultant, Fairfield Hospital, Melbourne, Australia.

Prevention

Immunization is only one approach to the control of disease, and when effective, it applies well to influenza. A Commonwealth Serum Laboratory product called influenza virus (sub-unit) vaccine 1971 is our standard vaccine. It is similar to some brands available in the United States. This vaccine was developed following the discovery by Webster and Laver[5] at the Australian National University that in experimental animals sodium deoxycholate abolished the toxicity of suspensions of influenza viruses without significant loss of antigenicity. The deoxycholate dissolves the lipids in the virus envelope while the surface antigens associated with infectivity are released in the form of sub-units. Influenza virus (sub-unit) vaccine is prepared by treating formalin inactivated virus vaccine with sodium deoxycholate. Our experience in organizing the first trials of this vaccine in infants with my colleagues, M.F. Warburton and Reuben Glass,[6] showed it to be non-reactogenic and antigenic. The same was found in adult volunteers.[7]

Composition of Vaccine

The vaccine contains 660 chick cell agglutinating (CCA) viral sub-units from the following strains of Influenza Virus Types A and B:

Influenza Virus Type A_2 Hong Kong Subtype (Strain A_2/NT/68)
Influenza Virus Type B (Strain B/Victoria/65)
Influenza Virus Type B (Strain B/Rome/67)

There is no doubt this vaccine causes fewer reactions than those previously used in Australia, and the only contra-indications are in a subject who is sensitive to egg albumin.

How Effective is the Vaccine?

Numerous trials, particularly by the United States Armed Forces Commission on Influenza, have demonstrated good protection against the natural disease. The World Health Organization (W.H.O.) believes that a suitable vaccine is indicated if a pandemic is threatened.

The warning system of the W.H.O. program functioned well with regards to the pandemic of A_2/Hong Kong influenza in 1968. Large amounts of vaccine were produced, but utilization was sub-optimal.[8]. When a second wave of the epidemic occurred one year later, there were 20,000 excess deaths in the United States, and a similar situation prevailed in Europe. Does this 1968-69 experience in the United States represent failure of antigens or failure of the strategy of immunization?

The answer is not just yes or no. Davenport and others[8] express the concept that community immunization programs could limit the spread of influenza virus.

Dr. A. A. Ferris,[8] former Director of the Virus Research Laboratory at Fairfield Hospital, reported that in the 1969 A_2/Hong Kong epidemic in Melbourne, over a two-month period, 96 patients were confirmed virologically, 84 patients by virus isolation, and 12 by serology alone. Twenty-eight of these 96 adult patients (29 per cent) had received the currently available vaccine. There were six deaths, four of whom had no pyogenic super-infections but died of classical influenza pneumonitis. None of the four persons who died had been vaccinated. These deaths were a rare and frightening phenomenon to us, but fortunately only occurred in a small number, and there were few deaths in children, with possible exception of a few cot deaths, in infants. The epidemic in 1969 was widespread, as shown in a sampling of 100 non-vaccinated blood donors — 52 per cent had antibody. This was similar to the 45 per cent found in the 1957 A_2 epidemic. There was quite a lot of very mild and subclinical A_2/Hong Kong influenza in Melbourne in 1969, yet in 1970, there was another epidemic with the same virus, with over 100 patients in hospital from whom a virus was isolated.

There is little doubt in the minds of clinicians that both in private and hospital practice, many lives were saved by the effective use of antibiotics during these influenza epidemics.

In Australia, the official view remains that vaccination with a current strain of vaccine is worthwhile, and gives up to 70 per cent

	Amantadine	Placebo	Totals
Number at risk	49	45	94
Number infected with A_2 during trial	17(35%)	20(45%)	37(40%)
Number of A_2 infections hospitalized	2(12%)	8(40%)	

TABLE 1

Results of a Trial of Amantadine to Prevent Influenza A Infection in Children

protection. In spite of this, some authorities doubt the value of vaccine, both for individual protection and for the slowing down of an epidemic. The reason for the failure of vaccine is perhaps that it does not produce local respiratory tract surface immunity (IgA).

It was shown in the amantadine trial in Melbourne that the 1968 A_2 Asian epidemic in children, although affecting 35 to 40 per cent, was a comparatively mild disease in that age group. Because of the dramatic pandemics of influenza in 1918, we are inclined to be too apprehensive about the expected epidemics, and the study in children in 1968 showed influenza to be no more serious than some other viral epidemics.

The National Health and Medical Research Council in Australia recommend vaccination in the following order of priority: (1) pregnant women; (2) children 1-5 years of age; (3) persons with chronic debilitating disease; and (4) persons over 65 years of age. (These persons should be immunized against influenza, and their immunity maintained with a yearly booster dose.) In addition, if an epidemic is threatened, vaccination should be performed on (1) persons in medical services and public utilities or communications; (2) persons in whom the incidence of infection is highest, namely aged 5-25 years; and (3) patients in nursing homes or chronic disease hospitals. Vaccine is not available on our National Health Scheme as a pharmaceutical benefit, except for pensioners.

There is no disquiet in Australia at the moment regarding the prospects of a severe epidemic of influenza B virus, but the manufacturer of the vaccine is alerting doctors, some of whom have started to immunize. There has been no direction from the public health authorities as yet, presumably awaiting the full reports of epidemics in the northern hemisphere.

Other Vaccines

Vaccination against influenza is at present still unsatisfactory, and live influenza vaccine may yet prove to be more effective. In the United Kingdom,[9] work has continued on the development and testing of live attenuated influenza A_2 strains for intra-nasal administration. The tissue IgA is raised by this method. Interferon production may make it more protective. The practical results so far are not very promising. However, in the USSR, 20-30 million doses annually of live influenza vaccine have been administered by the intra-nasal route. The oral route may also be effective.

Dr. Voroshilova[8] stated that enteroviruses are effective interferon inducers, and in field trials the incidence of influenza was reduced in groups who had received oral Type 1 polio vaccine.

A report by Dr. Woodhour[8] and associates suggested that Adjuvant 65 influenza vaccine was associated with increased anti-influenza antibody in nasal secretions. There is some doubt as to the oncogenicity of the mineral oil adjuvants.

Chemoprophylaxis with Amantadine

The important discovery of amantadine in 1964 has been well ventilated in this city and elsewhere.[10-12] A. A. Smorodintsev[8] and others showed in volunteers that amantadine was effective against the Hong Kong, as well as other strains of A_2. Unfortunately, it is not effective against influenza type B.

A double blind trial in children was carried out under my supervision in Melbourne at the start of the expected epidemic in 1968 of A_2

Asian influenza. The children selected were inmates of a child reception center, aged one to fourteen years. The children taking part had blood samples taken before the commencement of the drug. A second specimen was obtained ten weeks later, after cessation of amantadine. Viral, nasal and throat swabs were taken at the start and at intervals during the epidemic. Any infant or child who seemed sick was admitted to hospital, the decision being a "common sense" one, applying both to children on amantadine and on placebo.

Results

The figures seen in Table I are not statistically significant (p- .058). It was concluded, however, that our findings were consistent with the degree of protection shown in reported experimental trials in adults, and that amantadine is an effective prophylactic against A_2 influenza. In our experience the disease in children was not sufficiently severe to warrant its use routinely. It could be useful in debilitated patients. In most children infected the disease was mild and no special treatment was required. In more severe cases, although the symptoms may well have been due only to the virus, the accompanying pyogenic infection, which occurred in many cases, required an antibiotic.

Pyogenic Infection

One of the outstanding deficiences in our knowledge is the incidence of pyogenic complications in viral infection. It is known that 50 per cent of people carry potential pathogens in their nose, throat or ear. Pneumococcal infection is the commonest complicating infection and is adequately handled with penicillin and other drugs, such as lincomycin, erythromycin, and the cephalosporins. The same applies to streptococcal infection.

During the A_2 influenza epidemic in 1957 in Melbourne, a number of infants and older children in the community were infected with penicillin-resistant staphylococci, producing severe staphylococcal penumonia, and there were 20 deaths due to this cause. This calamitous experience has influenced our therapy to such an extent that since then one has used in severely ill patients erythromycin, lincomycin, or chloramphenicol. Tetracycline has been used a great deal in older children and adults. Both chloramphenicol and tetracycline can be combined with penicillin to make sure streptococci are well covered.

The purely viral pneumonia in children is seldom severe enough to be fatal. One infant died at the Royal Children's Hospital, and the post mortem findings were typical of viral pneumonia. The very severe cyanotic moist pneumonia, which occurred in four adults, defied all attempts of modern oxygen and resuscitation therapy.

Respiratory Syncytial Viral Infection

This virus is a frequent cause of severe respiratory infection in infants. Epidemics occur almost annually, and vaccines not only do not prevent the disease but can make it worse by means of a sensitivity phenomenon in the lungs.[13] Most cases are not helped by antibiotic therapy, and some authorities even condemn antibiotics in R.S.V. infection, but one fails to agree with this attitude because it is sometimes difficult to be certain if the infant has a purely viral condition. In therapy, oxygen is of paramount importance.

In Melbourne we have had an epidemic of R.S.V. with chiefly bronchiolitis in infants, every winter since 1960, with the exception of 1965. Last year there was a sudden epidemic in a neonatal nursery, but no deaths. Fluorescent antibody smear tests have been described for diagnosis by Gardner.[14]

Parainfluenza Virus — Prevention

Vaccines are under investigation for prevention of this virus infection. The importance of local nasal antibody has been stressed in regard to influenza, and probably also applies to parainfluenza.

These viruses, Types 1, 2, 3, are common causes of croup in children in Australia, and probably cause other respiratory syndromes in older patients. Diagnosis of the virus involved can be helped with fluorescent smear tests.[3]

Patients admitted to hospital are usually given antibiotics, and a broad spectrum approach with chloramphenicol is preferable in severe cases. In the care of the respiratory obstruction, steam tent therapy is standard. When indicated, intubation or tracheostomy is performed.

Adenovirus

Adenovirus is a common cause of respiratory infections, and the one currently present in Melbourne is Type 1. Occasionally, mixed viral infections such as measles and adeno virus Type 3, have produced a very sick patient with pneumonia.

Conclusion

The advanced techniques in the viral laboratories have shown the clinician there are at least 120 known respiratory viruses and strains. These can cause a variety of clinical syndromes. We now have a greater understanding of the mechanism of recurrent respiratory infection in children and an explanation why children are seldom well for lengthy periods.

Immunization is still worthy of consideration against influenza virus infection although the vaccines available are not ideal. Amantadine is an effective prophylactic against influenza A_2 virus. Antibiotics reduce morbidity and mortality due to pyogenic infections associated with these viral infections. Having practiced pediatrics before the antibiotic era, the author acknowledges the tremendous value of antibiotics in the care of children with respiratory infection.

REFERENCES

1. Stuart-Harris CH: Success and failure in human virus disease. Brit Med Jour 1:334, 1971.
2. Chanock RM, Parrott RH, Johnson KM, et al: Myxoviruses: Parainfluenza. Am Rev Resp Dis 88:Suppl 152, 1963.
3. Gardner PS, McQuillin J, McGuckin R, et al: Observations on clinical and immunofluorescent diagnosis of parainfluenza virus infections. Brit Med Jour 2:7, 1971.
4. Morbidity and Mortality. Vol 20, No 7, Feb 1971.
5. Webster RG and Laver WG: Influenza virus subunit vaccines: Immunogenicity and lack of toxicity of rabbits of ether- and detergent-disrupted virus. J Immunol 96:596 1966.
6. Warburton MF: Deoxycholate-split influenza vaccines. Bull Wld Hlth Org 41:639, 1969.
7. Duxbury AE, Hampson AW and Sievers JG: Antibody response in humans to deoxycholate-treated influenza virus vaccine. J Immunol 101:62, 1968.
8. Sandford JP: Rapporteurs International Conference on the Application of Vaccines against Viral, Rickettsial, and Bacterial Disease of Man. Pan American Health Organization, Dec 1970.
9. Editorial: Live influenza virus vaccines. Brit Med Jour 2:712, 1969.
10. Jackson GG, Muldoon RL and Akers LW: Serological evidence for prevention of influenza infection in volunteers by an anti-influenzal drug adamantadine hydrochloride. Antimicrobial and Chemotherapy, p 703, 1963.
11. Dawkins AT, Gallager LR, Togo Y, et al: Studies on induced influenza in man: II. Double-blind study designed to assess the prophylactic efficiency of an analogue of amantadine-hydrochloride. J Amer Med Ass 203:1095, 1968.
12. Oker-Blom N, Hovi T, Leinikki P, et al: Protection of man from natural infection with influenza A_2 Hong Kong virus by amantadine. Brit Med Jour 3:676, 1970.
13. Chanock RM: Control of acute mycoplasmal and viral respiratory tract disease. Science 169:248, 1970.
14. Gardner PS and McQuillin J: Application of immuno-fluorescent antibody technique in rapid diagnosis of respiratory syncytial virus infection. Brit Med Jour 3:340, 1968.

THE TREATMENT OF TUBERCULOSIS AND MYCOBACTERIAL PULMONARY DISEASE

● Continuing rapid advances in the diagnosis and treatment of tuberculosis require frequent review of this subject to assure proper management of the infected patient.

J. Woodrow Savacool, M.D.

Through the ages tuberculosis was known in various forms but was not well organized as an entity until the last two decades of the nineteenth century when its etiology was discovered and it became possible to observe its epidemiology. This led to efforts at prevention and control, which before long began to make inroads into its morbidity and mortality. Groups of persons other than physicians soon played an important role in dissemination of knowledge of the disease. The voluntary agencies which resulted provided a model for public efforts in many areas of disease control. In coming to Delaware to discuss tuberculosis treatment, one cannot help but refer to the role played by Delaware people in organizing the public for its part in publicity, public education and fund raising. The work of Emily Bissell and her Christmas Seal paved the way for the more recent efforts of people like Dr. Beatty whose memory is honored here and whose leadership in the anti-tuberculosis movement depended greatly on the groundwork laid in the beginning of the present century.

Supplementing the principles of isolation of active cases, hygienic treatment, collapse therapy and case finding, the discovery of specific antituberculosis drugs provided a final weapon which made the hope of disease eradication a possibility. In our country there are now large areas relatively free of tuberculosis. There is still, however, a large reservoir of persons who harbor the tubercle bacillus, and the relatively high prevalence of tuberculosis in crowded and urban areas attests to the fact that we still have a long way to go to achieve the goal. For this reason it is still important to use effectively the skills and knowledge which have made control procedures so rewarding during the past two decades. It is also important to realize that, in many parts of the world, the modern tools of control and treatment have not been effectively applied and tuberculosis continues to be a major health problem.

The availability of effective drugs has produced a change in the logistics of tuberculosis treatment. Whereas formerly long-term isolation was a major need, most patients now show early conversion to non-infectious status, limiting both hospital stay and loss of time from work. Evidence has accumulated that bed rest, formerly the mainstay of treatment, is unnecessary and may be detrimental once the toxic phase of the disease is controlled. Surgical procedures, which were first brought within the limits of safety by anti-tuberculous

Dr. Savacool is Clinical Associate Professor of Medicine, Jefferson Medical College, Thomas Jefferson University.

drugs, are now rarely needed since experience has shown that residual lesions, including cavities, constitute less of a threat than was formerly believed. The need for specialized institutions therefore has diminished, and the need for better general hospital care of tuberculous patients, outpatient and laboratory facilities has increased. Recent recommendations of the American Thoracic Society Ad Hoc Committee on Quality Care for Tuberculosis[1] include availability of high quality medical care, an effective regimen of chemotherapy, microbiologic services, social and economic aid, and effective teaching of patients. Persons in whom the diagnosis of tuberculosis is suspected or confirmed are properly begun with treatment in general hospitals with the hope of continuing as outpatients once the immediate goals have been met and effective drug treatment initiated.[2,3]

Diagnosis

The fact that tuberculosis is often suspected for reasons other than presentation with specific symptoms at times requires that treatment begin without microbial confirmation. Collection of specimens for diagnosis should be carried out promptly with sputum smears and cultures and, in persons who cannot produce adequate specimens, by induction with saline or propylene glycol aerosol inhalation. Bronchoscopy for diagnosis and collection of secretions, pleural biopsy and fluid examination in cases of pleural effusion constitute other methods of procuring specimens for smear and culture. Once such efforts have been made and clinical judgment dictates tuberculosis as a presumptive diagnosis, treatment should be instituted. From there on, the diagnosis may be revised at any time new evidence is presented. There is a constant need to be critical of one's judgment so that treatment can be altered in accord with new developments.

The finding of acid-fast bacilli on smear must always be supplemented by typical growth on standard culture media. In every new culture, sensitivity studies for standard drugs are necessary even though in the United States 94 to 98% should prove sensitive.[4] Cultures not sensitive to primary drugs should

automatically be studied for sensitivity to secondary drugs, and under most circumstances treatment should be limited to primary drugs until such reports are available. Since the laboratory procedures for secondary drug sensitivity are specialized, they should be carried out in a few central, specially oriented laboratories where skills have been properly developed. When cultures reveal mycobacteria not typical of tuberculosis, an alternative diagnosis and plan for treatment must be made.

Standard Treatment

It has long been my practice to begin treatment with three drugs, streptomycin 1 gm intramuscularly daily, isoniazid and aminosalicylic acid. Streptomycin is well tolerated generally except in older persons in whom vestibular symptoms are prone to occur early. Isoniazid is given in doses averaging 5 mg per kilo per day and constitutes the mainstay of antituberculous treatment. Para-aminosalicylic acid is mildly tuberculostatic, but its principal use is prevention of isoniazid resistance. The dose is 12 gm daily as the sodium salt, but it may be modified in the presence of mild gastrointestinal symptoms. About 80% of persons can tolerate this drug in standard dose with good medical and nursing instruction. In persons with extensive or acutely symptomatic disease the program is now preferably modified to employ ethambutol instead of PAS, thus providing three potent drugs from the beginning. When after the first several months sensitivity studies indicate that the bacilli are normally sensitive to primary drugs, streptomycin is usually no longer needed; and, providing clinical improvement is adequate, INH and PAS or ethambutol may then be continued for the long term.[5] The principal indices of clinical improvement must always be the x-ray and bacteriologic findings. It is not unusual for symptoms to diminish so rapidly that within three or four weeks sputum is no longer obtainable by usual means and recourse must be had to induced sputum or gastrics for bacteriologic control. It is our practice unequivocally to advise patients to stop smoking at the beginning of treatment of any pulmonary disease ("People with trouble in their lungs should not smoke").

If this is observed, it also tends to increase the rapidity of symptom disappearance.

Treatment of new cases of pulmonary tuberculosis thus should prove excellent when circumstances can be controlled. In several series, tubercle bacilli have been eliminated from the sputum in 90 to 95% of newly diagnosed patients within six months. The relapse rate among such persons should be very low providing the treatment program is completed as planned.

Between the primary and secondary drugs is ethambutol, studied experimentally for a long time and released by the FDA late in 1967. It is an excellent antituberculous drug and may replace PAS as an adjunct to isoniazid. At present experience with it is increasing, patient acceptance is better than for PAS, and when properly used its potential toxicity can readily be controlled. The proper dose is now 25 mg per kilo given in one daily dose for two months, after which the dose is reduced to 15 mg per kilo per day. In addition to the usual medical follow-up, eye examinations for visual acuity, color vision and visual fields are needed. In present dosage the incidence of ill effects is small and the early ones reversible. It is likely that the combination of INH and ethambutol will be increasingly frequently employed as a basic antituberculous treatment plan.

The group of drugs generally included among those regarded as "secondary" antituberculous ones are those possessing more limited antituberculous potential or more frequent and serious side effects. They may be listed as follows: cycloserine, pyrizinamide, ethionamide, kanamycin, viomycin and capreomycin. The skillful employment of secondary drugs requires careful attention to bacterial sensitivity patterns, good laboratory control and the potential side effects of each agent singly and in combination. The specific side effects of each agent are beyond the scope of this presentation, but in general a combination of three or more drugs is employed against bacteria resistant to the primary agents. In this country the need for secondary drugs is most commonly encountered among alcoholics, recalcitrant patients or those who have for other reasons had capricious or in-

terrupted treatment or who have genetically determined inactivation of isoniazid. It is important to emphasize that resistance of bacteria to isoniazid is encouraged by injudicious or sporadic use in the presence of active disease especially under unsupervised circumstances.[6,7]

Many attempts have been made to determine the optimum time for total drug treatment. In some individuals with prompt bacteriologic conversion and x-ray retrogression, one has the impression that the battle is over early. However, treatment must continue well beyond the time required for stability. The Medical Research Council of Great Britain has established 24 months as the optimum period of basic therapy. I agree with this general program. In cases where bacteriologic conversion has been slow and much residual disease persists, uninterrupted drug treatment should be continued for at least three years and isoniazid may be extended for many months. In persons with complications of pneumoconiosis, alcoholism, duodenal ulcer and diabetes, isoniazid may be continued indefinitely for prophylaxis of relapse. Wherever treatment with secondary drugs has been successful, it has become standard procedure to continue that program for 24 months, and thereafter isoniazid may be extended for its preventive effect.

In any retreatment program, again the conversion of sputum and rehabilitation of the patients will depend mainly upon the disciplined completion of the planned program. Many reports are available which show a high percentage of patients experiencing sputum conversion even without rifampin. Using rifampin, ethambutol and capreomycin, Finnish investigators have reported 30 of 31 patients converted to negative in spite of previously having been classified as incurable because of drug resistance and drug intolerance.[8] There is thus much variation depending on the circumstances and previous treatment. There will no doubt continue to be a "hard core" of older persons with adverse factors in whom control will be difficult.[9]

An exciting new prospect is the imminent availability of rifampin, an antibiotic developed in Italy as rifamycin B obtained from culture media of *Streptomyces mediterranei.* Originally described in glowing terms in early European studies as effective against drug-resistant tubercle bacilli and atypical mycobacteria without toxic or side effects, it is now evident that these claims have been too sweeping. However, the recent report of controlled experimental studies carried out by the United States Public Health Service[10] suggests that rifampin can be safely employed and that isoniazid and rifampin may be the best combination of drugs for primary treatment of tuberculosis to date. 95% of patients in that study with far advanced cavitary disease showed elimination of tubercle bacilli from the sputum in 16 to 20 weeks of treatment. Although its place in treatment remains to be established, one may state now that rules similar to those governing other antituberculous agents must be applied to rifampin therapy. It may well achieve pre-eminent status as a first line drug when combined with isoniazid, but until further clinical experience has evolved, its major usefulness will probably be as a secondary drug combined with at least two other effective agents.[11] Two characteristics may be mentioned: (1) Its mode of action is by inhibition of DNA-dependent RNA polymerase activity in susceptible cells;[12] (2) it is highly concentrated in the liver and especially the bile, which may account for its tendency toward hepatitis-like toxicity in some individuals, especially those with other stigmata of hepato-biliary disease.

In present treatment programs, rifampin is given in the single daily dose of 600 mg one hour before breakfast.

Drug Reactions

Most persons tolerate antituberculous therapy well. However, the occurrence of tuberculosis in persons who are older, have other diseases and may be alcoholic increases the need for vigilance with respect to any drug treatment and especially combination drug treatment. These multiple factors have made more than usually difficult the evaluation of reactions to drugs, especially isoniazid. Hepatic toxicity from isoniazid and PAS in older persons has generally been attributed to PAS,

but it is now known that a form of liver disease may occur with isoniazid alone.[13] As a general rule, however, reactions to isoniazid are mild, and when medical supervision is good, early detection and usually cancellation of the drug will prevent serious complications. Further, if hepatic and enzymatic changes do not occur during the first two months of treatment, prolonged use of the drug is regarded as safe. In view of the publicity accorded isoniazid reactions during prophylaxis of a Washington, D. C. group of exposed individuals, the United States Public Health Service and the American Thoracic Society[14] have reaffirmed the desirability of continuing well established therapeutic and prophylactic programs albeit with increased vigilance. It may be stated, however, that in any prophylactic program where persons present multiple factors which could contribute to reactions, one might judiciously evaluate the risk and conclude that in such persons the risk of drug prophylaxis might well outweigh the risk of tuberculosis. In older epileptics, for example, who have only moderate tuberculin reactions with negative chest x-rays, we have not given isoniazid prophylaxis. Pyridoxine for prevention of peripheral neuropathy has some status and is probably needed for older persons and those with other risks, but in younger individuals with standard doses of isoniazid, the need for it has not been established. It has become customary for some health departments to include 5 mg of pyridoxine in 100 mg tablets of isoniazid. When larger doses are employed or in special situations, 50 to 100 mg of pyridoxine should be given daily.

Ill effects from PAS are common, especially gastrointestinal symptoms. Usually it is possible to adjust the dose and timing of the medication to overcome them, but when such side effects are persistent, one should look for hepatic toxicity or other evidence of idiosyncrasy or hypersensitivity and begin an alternative drug program.

Streptomycin is generally well tolerated. Vestibular symptoms may occur early and require that the drug be stopped since, rarely, progression to hearing loss may occur. Drug fever and skin lesions are readily detected and also require cancellation. Persons with renal failure concentrate the drug unduly, and dosage must be adjusted or treatment changed.

In the past the disability relative to the treatment of tuberculosis and its infectious nature have been among its most devastating effects. Middle-aged persons who have been out of work for months or years have found it virtually impossible to return to gainful employment after such long lapses. Now the patient can usually return to work after a brief and intensive period of medication and teaching. Changes in careers are no longer necessary except when the problem is complicated. Moderately strenuous physical activity is permissible with regular hours of employment. Once cough and sputum and x-ray findings show significant improvement, it may reasonably be concluded that the program is successful, and the patient may return to work. It is often necessary, however, to overcome the traditional resistance on the part of personnel directors, physicians and nurses. In those cases where ideal circumstances do not pertain, duration of disability may be limited by rehabilitative programs which must begin during rather than at the end of the active treatment period.

Not all persons with active tuberculosis do well. Some already have other illnesses, others fail to cooperate, or special circumstances develop. Persistent cavities, residual from tuberculous ones, may remain in spite of sputum conversion. These are referred to as "open negative."[15] We have now observed more than one hundred of these, and it is possible to state that most of them do well provided bacteriologic conversion was prompt and clinical recovery otherwise complete. About 10% of those who do poorly develop fungus diseases, including mycetomata, in the cavities. These fungus balls are most commonly due to aspergillosis, and the principal hazard is hemorrhage. A few of the "open negative" relapse with recurrent positive sputum, and some show progression toward bullous emphysema which in itself may become disabling. In spite of these occasional complications, however, surgical resection of portions of lungs bearing such residual cavities is no longer generally recommended. There is a place, how-

ever, for surgical resection in a few special cases, especially in young persons and in those for whom it may not be possible to carry on appropriate follow-up treatment.

Mycobacteriosis

Although the atypical mycobacteria have been observed for many years, mainly the chromogenic ones, their clinical status has been enigmatic. Since we have specific drug treatment for tuberculosis, however, it has become important to establish the status of these mycobacteria as clearly as possible so that specific treatment might be used where applicable and undue concern over the less important bacteria be avoided. Some exist only as saprophytes and as such may be found in the presence of other pulmonary diseases without etiological significance; others are definitely etiologic. It has been possible in recent years to classify and evaluate the roles of these organisms to some degree. It is now preferable to regard disease produced by atypical mycobacteria as mycobacteriosis which, though exhibiting properties similar to those of tuberculosis, yet constitutes a somewhat different disease epidemiologically and therapeutically. An important distinction is that transmission of atypical mycobacteria from person to person has not been established. Although some strains are common in nature, the mode of human acquisition of the organisms is unknown. The important ones from the standpoint of human pulmonary disease have been grouped as follows:

Group I   Photochromogenic:
                 M. kansasii
Group II   Scotochromogenic:
                 M. scrofulaceum
Group III Nonchromogenic:
                 M. intracellulare
Group IV Rapid growers:
                 M. fortuitum

It is relatively uncommon to make a primary diagnosis of mycobacteriosis. Most commonly the diagnosis of tuberculosis is made because of x-ray findings and the presence of acid-fast bacilli on smears. Treatment with drugs is then begun, and only when the response of the patient is unusual or the cultures are reported does one suspect or prove that the process is not tuberculosis. A change in therapy may then be made depending upon the circumstances. It is important to acknowledge that it is not possible to differentiate the mycobacterioses from tuberculosis by x-ray or histological methods. The clinical course of mycobacteriosis is commonly characterized by a waxing and waning of lesions as shown by x-ray. This is especially so if the organisms are resistant to the treatment which has been instituted. The indolence of the lesions and the lack of communicability also remove some of the urgency about the management. Generally patients may work, and it is preferable to permit drug treatment or treatment change to await results of sensitivity studies. This again underlines the importance of distinguishing *M. tuberculosis* from the atypical mycobacteria and carrying through with all possible microbiological identification procedures including drug sensitivity studies.

I have collected 23 cases for observation although we have seen many more in whom studies are not complete. Of the 23, 13 are due to *M. kansasii* (Group I), 8 to *M. intracellulare* (Group III), two to Group II. In one case there were two species of atypical mycobacteria cultured and in two cases, three species. Generally those with several species have been more ill and have had other pulmonary problems. We have also experienced the occurrence of mycobacteriosis in persons previously having had a documented diagnosis of tuberculosis.

Several guidelines have emerged. In persons with previously established pulmonary disease such as pneumoconiosis, bronchiectasis or emphysema, it is relatively more common to have saprophytic mycobacteria which often belong to Group II or IV. In primary mycobacteriosis, the usual pathogens are *M. kansasii* and *M. intracellulare*, especially the Battey-Avium-Swine strain. Also generally *M. kansasii* may respond to ethambutol and cycloserine in combination although some strains are sensitive to streptomycin. If the latter is used, it should be given daily. The Battey strain is less likely to respond to drugs, and only occasionally are members of this

group responsive to rifampin. Since some question the comparability of *in vitro* studies with clinical usefulness, it has been proposed that atypical infections might best be treated with combinations of ethambutol, cycloserine and ethionamide while awaiting the availability of rifampin. However, there is much to be said for not undertaking any new treatment program until one has the guidance of sensitivity studies since progression of the disease is usually slow and interrupted. It should be mentioned in passing that the penicillins and erythromycin have proven effective against certain strains of mycobacteria, but the place of these agents remains to be established. We have had one experience where penicillin in large doses appeared clinically effective against a disease produced by a strain of Group IV organisms. Also it has been shown, especially where disease is localized within one lobe, surgical excision may be the preferred treatment.[16] This is limited by the fact that these infections often occur in older persons in whom the surgical risk may be inordinate.

How much of a problem is mycobacteriosis? Our experience shows that one case is discovered for each ten or twelve new cases of tuberculosis, but statistics are difficult to clarify. It is not clear whether the disease is increasing in frequency or not, but the relative importance of these organisms has increased with the decreased incidence of new cases of tuberculosis. It is sufficiently important that we need to think of it in the differential diagnosis of chronic pulmonary disease generally.

Summary

1. Tuberculosis diagnosis and treatment are becoming increasingly the responsibility of practicing physicians and general hospitals.

2. Hospitalization now should be intended primarily for confirmation of diagnosis, initiation of specific treatment and teaching the patient.

3. Although the treatment of newly diagnosed tuberculosis is disarmingly simple, treatment failures and retreatment problems involving resistant tubercle bacilli

require care, precision and multiple drug therapy with attendant risk of intolerance and idiosyncrasy. Every effort must be made to assure success the first time.

4. Specificity of microbiological diagnosis is of major importance in management of all diseases produced by mycobacteria.

5. Rifampin may well prove an important new weapon for primary treatment once its indications and limitations have been established.

REFERENCES

1. Standards for Tuberculosis Treatment in the 1970's: A Statement of the Ad Hoc Committee on Quality Care for Tuberculosis. Am Rev Resp Dis 102:992, 1970.
2. Guidelines for the General Hospital in the Admission and Care of Tuberculous Patients. Ad Hoc Committee of American Thoracic Society. Am Rev Resp Dis 99:631, 1969.
3. Fahy A: This big city pushes clinic care for TB. Bulletin National Tuberculosis and Respiratory Disease Association, March 1971.
4. Hobby GL, Johnson PM, Boytar-Papirnyck V. et al: Primary drug resistance: A continuing study of tubercle in a veteran population within the United States. VI. Initial observations on the incidence of resistance to rifampin and ethambutol. Am Rev Resp Dis 99:777, 1969.
5. Johnston RF and Hopewell PC: Chemotherapy of pulmonary tuberculosis. Ann Int Med 70:359, 1969.
6. Drug Resistant Tuberculosis: A Review of the World Situation. Tubercle 50, Supplement 2, 1969.
7. The Chemotherapy of Tuberculosis in Developing Countries. Tubercle 49, Supplement, 1969.
8. Hellstrom PE and Repo UK: Scand Jour Resp Dis Supplement, 1969.
9. Steiner M, Chaves A. Lyons HA, et al: Primary drug-resistant tuberculosis. NEJM 283:1353, 1970.
10. Newman R, Doster B, Murray FJ, et al: Rifampin in initial treatment of pulmonary tuberculosis. Am Rev Resp Dis 103:461, 1971.
11. Vall-Spinosa A and Lester W: Rifampin in the treatment of drug-resistant mycobacterium tuberculosis infections. NEJM 283:616, 1970.
12. Editorial: Colloquium on RNA polymerase. Nature (London) 224:10, 1969.
13. Scharer L and Smith JP: Serum transaminase elevations and other hepatic abnormalities in patients receiving isoniazid. Ann Int Med 71:1113, 1969.
14. Isoniazid-associated Liver Disease Meeting of the Ad Hoc Advisory Committee on Isoniazid and Liver Disease (Report #4), March 19, 1971. To be published.
15. Corpe RF and Blalock FA: Continuing study of patients with "open negative" status at Battey State Hospital. Am Rev Resp Dis 98:954, 1968.
16. Thong K: Resection in patients with atypical pulmonary tuberculosis. Med J Aust 748-751, 1969.

※ ※ ※

RECENT TRENDS IN THE MANAGEMENT OF

HEPATIC ABSCESS

● An undiagnosed hepatic abscess is invariably fatal. A high index of suspicion should lead to the necessary diagnostic laboratory and radiologic procedures to permit specific surgical and antibiotic therapy.

WILLIAM A. ALTEMEIER, M.D.*

The obscure nature of hepatic abscesses with their lack of prominent localizing signs and their association with other more dominant diseases has frequently resulted in prolonged diagnostic delays or failures until serious complications or death occurred.[1-7] In our experience, hepatic abscess has been a life-threatening disease, and failure to diagnose and adequately drain these abscesses has invariably been fatal. Antibiotic therapy has been shown to be a valuable adjunctive agent in the pre- and post-operative control of these infections, but it has not prevented death when abscesses were not drained.[8,9] The recent utilization of new diagnostic techniques, however, has greatly improved the treatment and reduced the mortality of patients with this serious infection.[10-14] Earlier diagnosis and improved localization of hepatic abscesses have become possible preoperatively through the introduction and the use of radioisotope liver scans and arteriograms of the celiac axis. As a result, earlier and effective surgical drainage has thus become possible, and this has proven to be of considerable importance in the patients' survival. In contrast to previous reports, the last nine cases seen by the author during the past two years have been correctly diagnosed preoperatively and drained successfully with no mortality.

To obtain a better knowledge of the nature of these infections and to study the availability and effectiveness of the methods of their diagnosis and treatment, a study of all patients with hepatic abscesses who were seen on the Surgical Services of the University of Cincinnati Medical Center during the past 16 years has been made.

Materials and Methods

Cases of diagnosed and clearly documented liver abscess which were seen during the 16 years from January 1955 through January 1971 were included in this study. This case material was from the four hospitals of the University of Cincinnati Hospital Group: Cincinnati General Hospital, Cincinnati Veterans Administration Hospital, Christian R. Holmes Hospital, and Cincinnati Children's Hospital. In each instance the pathology was substantiated at operation or necropsy. Example of pyogenic, amoebic, echinococcal, and actinomycotic abscesses were found. In all, a total of 68 cases were studied, 61 being classified as pyogenic, four amoebic, two fungal and one echinococcal.

For purposes of comparison and discussion of the incidence, etiology, pathogenesis, diagnostic problems, effectiveness of treatment, morbidity, and mortality, this study was divided into three periods of five, five, and six years. (Table I) Further subdivision of the patients into two groups was based upon whether or not surgical intervention with

Dr. Altemeier is Professor of Surgery and Chairman of the Department, University of Cincinnati.

*Work described was supported in part by U.S.P.H.S. Grant 5-POI-GM-15428 and U.S. Army Contract DA-49-193-MD-2531.

(68 Cases)				
Period	Pyogenic	Amoebic	Fungal	Echinococcal	Total
1955 - 1959	22	0	1	0	23
1960 - 1964	19	0	0	0	19
1965 - 1970	20	4	1	1	26
Total	61	4	2	1	68

TABLE I

INCIDENCE AND ETIOLOGY
OF LIVER ABSCESSES

drainage of the abscesses was or would have been beneficial. (Table II) The liver abscesses in 41 of the patients were found to have been amenable to surgical drainage (Group I) and 27 were not (Group II). The abscesses found in Group I were 1.5 cm or greater in diameter and were noted to be either solitary and discrete, or confluent. (Table III). The largest abscess contained 1200 cc of pus and measured 15 cm in diameter. Evidence of septicemia and multiple abscesses in other organs was usually absent in patients of this type. Those in Group II, however, were smaller and in some instances microscopic, being almost invariably multiple, and usually associated with septicemia documented by positive blood cultures. (Table IV) Abscesses in other organs were frequently present and multiple in this group.

Other categories studied were age, sex, race, microbial etiology, pathogenesis, clinical features, laboratory data, x-ray examinations, liver scans, and arteriograms. Attention was focused particularly on those factors which led to increased mortality and morbidity such as delay or failure in diagnosis, inadequate surgical operations, poor bacteriological culture techniques, or failure to detect and manage complications and associated diseases.

Results

Incidence The numbers of patients with liver abscesses occurring in the three periods

of this study were 23, 19, and 26. (Table I) There were 34 patients with pyogenic abscesses amenable to surgical drainage (Group I), and their incidence was evenly distributed over the sixteen-year period. (Table II) The four cases of amoebic abscess and one of *echinococcus* disease all occurred in the most recent six-year period. Of the 27 cases not amenable to surgery, 13 were in the first five-year period, eight in the second, and six in the last six years.

Age The youngest patient in the total series was 12 days of age and the oldest 90 years of age, the average being 47.6 years. The majority of the patients in the total group were found in the first, seventh, and eighth decades. In the operable group these peaks were not evident, and almost equal numbers of cases occurred in each decade from the fourth to the eighth inclusive.

Sex and Race There were 48 males and 20 females. Forty-three patients were Caucasian and 25 Negro. The sex and race ratios did not vary in Group I and Group II from the total series.

Location and Nature of the Abscesses Of the 68 cases, 36 involved a single lobe, while 30 were bilateral and multiple. In two small abscesses identified at autopsy, the location was not specified. Of the 41 patients considered to be amenable to surgery, 26 had single abscesses and 23 of these were located in the

(Group I)				
Period	Pyogenic	Amoebic	Fungal	Echinococcal	Total
1955 - 1959	9	0	1	0	10
1960 - 1964	11	0	0	0	11
1965 - 1970	14	4	1	1	20
Total	34	4	2	1	41

TABLE II

INCIDENCE AND ETIOLOGY
OF LIVER ABSCESSES
AMENABLE TO SURGICAL
INTERVENTION

TABLE III

LOCATION OF LIVER ABSCESSES IN CASES
AMENABLE TO SURGICAL INTERVENTION

(Group I)

Type	Right Lobe	Left Lobe	Bilateral	Total
Single (26 Cases)	23	3	—	26
Multiple (15 Cases)	2	4	9	15
Total	25	7	9	41

right lobe. (Table III) The last case seen was of special interest since it was characterized by an irregular coalesced abscess in the right lobe and multiple smaller abscesses 1-3 mm in diameter throughout both lobes. Of the 27 patients with bilateral and multiple abscesses, 21 fell into the non-operable group. (Table V)

Clinical Picture In Group I, the most commonly noted signs were temperature elevations in 95 percent, hepatomegaly in 51 percent, abdominal tenderness in 51 percent, and jaundice in 28 percent. Abnormal chest findings contiguous to the area of the hepatic disease were noted in 20 percent of the cases. The majority of the temperature elevations ranged between 102 and 106 F. Equivalent numbers of patients had elevations between 104 and 106 F. as had elevations between 102 and 104 F. The typical spiking temperature course observed is well illustrated in Figure I. Abdominal pain was the most common symptom noted. Chills were noted in only nine cases or 22 percent. (Table VI)

The clinical features of the cases in Group II with multiple abscesses not amenable to sur-

TABLE IV

LOCATION OF LIVER ABSCESSES IN CASES
NOT AMENABLE TO SURGICAL INTERVENTION

(Group II)

Type	Right Lobe	Left Lobe	Bilateral	Total
Single	1	1	—	4*
Multiple	1	—	22	23
Total	2	1	22	27

*In two small abscesses identified at autopsy, location was not specified.

gery were usually related to the non-specific signs of sepsis or to a remote primary disease process.

Laboratory Data The average white cell count for the 68 patients was 20,900 with the highest count being 61,600 and the lowest being 2,500. Patients with known blood disorders such as leukemia were not included in the tabulation. The average hemoglobin recorded was 11.4 grams and the average hematocrit was 33.4 percent.

Of special interest were the abnormal serum albumin, alkaline phosphatase, and bilirubin liver function studies. The serum albumin was 3.0 grams percent or less in 76 percent of the cases, and the alkaline phosphatase was elevated in 74 percent. Although bromsulphalein retention was measured in only ten patients, it was abnormal in all but one. Fifteen of 41 patients with operable abscesses had an elevated bilirubin. Thirteen of these had associated disease of the extrahepatic bile ducts and elevated alkaline phosphatase levels. The SGOT and SGPT measurements were normal in most instances.

Radiologic Examinations X-ray examinations were of only limited value in the diagnosis of hepatic abscesses. Intravenous or oral cholecystograms, obtained in eight patients, did not produce visualization of the gall bladder or biliary tree in any. In five cases marked jaundice was present, however, and the presence of biliary tract disease was subsequently confirmed in each of these.

X-rays of the chest were found to be abnormal in 19 instances and were related to the position and size of the abscesses present. (Figure II) In eight patients the appropriate diaphragm was elevated, and in 12 cases pleural effusion or pulmonary infiltrate was noted adjacent to the hepatic disease. The chest film appeared to be completely normal in ten cases, however.

An upper gastrointestinal series was performed in nine patients and was found to be abnormal in eight. A mass lesion was suggested in the liver in one case in which an abscess of the left lobe enlarged the liver sufficiently to compress the lesser curvature of

125

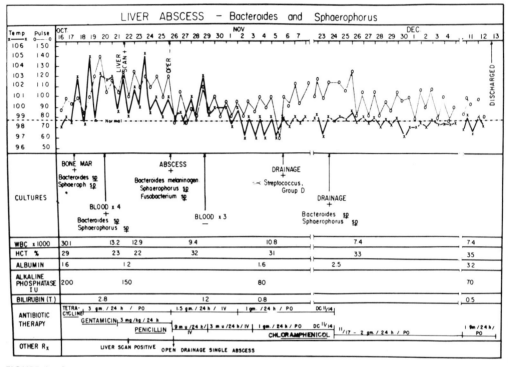

FIGURE I   Septic course of 44-year-old male patient with obscure liver abscess and eight-week history. Liver scan revealed large defect in lateral aspect of right lobe. (Reprinted from Archives of Surgery, Vol. 101, page 258, August 1970.)

the stomach.

Hepatic Radioisotope Scans Liver scans have been of great diagnostic value in demonstrating and localizing hepatic abscesses. In all instances but one, abnormal scans were obtained in those patients in which it was used. The changes were subsequently shown to represent suppurative hepatic disease. (Figure III) In only one patient, proven to have numerous small hepatic abscesses less than 2 cm in diameter, was the scan reported to be negative. The majority of the scans performed in our patients utilized the sulfur colloid, technetium Tc99m, and the Photogamma II or Photogamma III scintillation cameras.

Selective Arteriography Arteriography has also been employed in all of the most recent cases. It has been of value in confirming mod-

erate- and large-sized defects demonstrated by liver scans. Such areas suspected of representing an abscess were proven to be avascular by the selective arteriogram. (Figure IV)

Etiology Specific culture information was available from 21 of the 34 operable pyogenic abscesses. *Escherichia coli* was grown in pure culture from eight (42%) of the 19 cases over the 15-year period. In the past five years, more sophisticated bacteriologic studies have been made, and anaerobic organisms including the anaerobic *Streptococcus, Bacteroides sp., Sphaerophorus sp.,* or *Fusobacterium sp.* were cultured without associated aerobic growth in eight instances. In these cases the cultures would otherwise have been negative or had been previously reported as negative. During the past three years, anaerobes have been isolated exclusively in all cases except for two

126

abscesses in which *E. coli* was grown in pure culture and one case in which *Streptococcus viridans* was cultured in association with the anaerobic *Streptococcus.*

Amoebae were not cultured but were identified on smear from the wound drainage in one instance. In three of the four cases a positive hemagglutination test was obtained to support the diagnosis.

Actinomyces israelli was cultured from each case suspected of being fungal in nature. Biopsies of the hepatic abscess wall also demonstrated the *Actinomyces.*

The larvae with scolices and hooklets of *Echinococcus granulosus* were identified in the case of *echinococcus* disease seen.

Pathogenesis In the Group I patients with pyogenic abscesses of the liver amenable to surgical drainage, direct hepatic involvement by a primary disease served as the portal of entry in 11 cases. Of these, cholangitis was believed to be dominant in eight patients and pylephlebitis in three. Septicemia was the only apparent source of hepatic infection in two other cases, and in ten the sources of infection were not apparent, making the etiology obscure. This latter group was therefore classified as cryptogenic.

In Group II patients, septicemias were noted to be the dominant process in approximately two-thirds of the cases. The sources in four

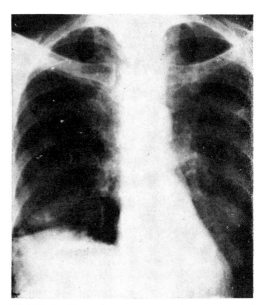

FIGURE 2 Chest roentgenogram showing marked elevation of the right diaphragm and changes above and below diaphragm caused by large liver abscess, which had perforated to produce an extensive subphrenic abscess.

were believed to be cholangitic, in three the liver was involved directly, and in four the mechanisms were uncertain.

Associated Diseases Various diseases associated with pyogenic liver abscess appeared to be of considerable clinical significance. Disease of the extrahepatic biliary tree was the most frequent associated illness in 13 of the 34 patients with surgically significant hepatic abscesses. An obstructive component due to calculi or malignant disease including carcinoma of the pancreas, gallbladder, or bile ducts was present in nine. Five had abscesses involving the hepatic substance in the area of the gall bladder bed related either to empyema or a pericholecystic abscess.

Seven liver abscesses developed in areas of previously existing intrahepatic disease. Hepatic polycystic disease was encountered with infection in three of these, having developed in the intrahepatic cysts. In three other cases, the abscesses were related to metastatic carcinoma with necrosis and secondary infection.

TABLE V
CLINICAL SIGNS AND SYMPTOMS
IN PATIENTS WITH LIVER ABSCESSES
AMENABLE TO SURGERY
(Group I — 41 Patients)

Signs and Symptoms	Patients	Percent
Temperature Elevation	39	95
Abdominal Pain	25	61
Anorexia	22	53
Hepatomegaly	21	51
Abdominal Tenderness	21	51
Fever	18	43
Jaundice	12	28
Pulmonary Signs	8	20
Chills	9	22
Vomiting	6	14
Respiratory Symptoms	5	12

TABLE VI
DISEASES ASSOCIATED WITH PYOGENIC
ABSCESSES AMENABLE TO SURGERY
34 PATIENTS

Biliary Tract Disease		13
Inflammatory Disease	9	
Malignant Disease	4	
Intrahepatic Disease		7
Polycystic Disease of the Liver	3	
Metastatic Carcinoma	3	
Tuberculous Involvement	1	
Extrahepatic Extrabiliary Disease		14
Pneumonia	3	
Peritonitis	1	
Probable Pre-existing Appendicitis	1	
Chronic Pancreatitis	1	
Diverticulitis with Abscess	2	
Subphrenic and Interloop Abscesses	1	
Regional Enteritis	1	
Ulcerative Proctitis Acute Hemorrhagic Pancreatitis	1	
Pneumonia-Meningitis-Septicemia	1	
Urinary Tract Infection	1	
Total		34

Two of these primary malignancies were of colon origin and one of the lung. One case appeared to have resulted from the extension of a tuberculous empyema into the dome of the liver. In the 12 cases, extrahepatic extrabiliary diseases were associated with the suppurative hepatic disease.

The prominent disease processes associated with the abscesses not amenable to surgery were often extraperitoneal and related to the suppurative hepatic disease most often by septicemia alone.

Of the eleven children, only three had abscesses amenable to surgical drainage. In one the abscesses were complications of a severe regional enteritis. This rare complication of regional enteritis has been previously described.[15] In the other two children the etiology was obscure. Of the remaining children, three had associated lymphoblastic leukemia, two were premature infants with associated infection, one had extrahepatic biliary

atresia, and three others succumbed to a septicemia originating from an extrahepatic source.

Among the other associated diseases was diabetes mellitus found in approximately 15 percent of the patients in the total series, and septicemia occurred in one-third of these. The association of diabetes mellitus and hepatic abscess has been noted previously.[16] The septicemia was believed to be a complication of the hepatic abscess in most of the patients with lesions adaptable to surgical drainage,[17] and septicemia occurred in over half of these patients (56 percent).

Complications The complications which were recognized are listed in Table VII. Seventeen cases in which septicemia was believed to be a complication of the hepatic abscess are included. Four abscesses ruptured into the subphrenic space without further extension, and each of these was pyogenic in nature. Four others extended into the pleural cavity to produce an associated empyema, three of these being amoebic and one pyogenic. Two perforated into the peritoneal cavity with resultant generalized peritonitis. Both of these involved necrotic metastic carcinomas.

The patient with echinococcal disease of the liver leaked from the cysts preoperatively, and at surgery daughter cysts were noted on the surface of the liver and adjacent hepatic flexure.

One amoebic abscess drained itself spontaneously through the diaphragm, lung, and bronchial tree. The patient with regional enteritis developed a recurrent abscess approximately one month following her initial drainage procedure. (Figure V) Another suffered a massive pulmonary embolism and expired in the postoperative period.

Surgical Procedures The surgical approach in all cases but one was transabdominal, the position of the incision depending upon the suspected or demonstrated location of the abscess. In most cases the incision was a right subcostal one. When possible, drainage was performed extraperitoneally. This was frequently impossible, however, because of the lack of adhesion between the liver and the

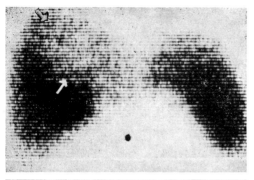

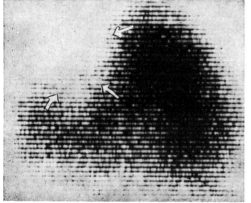

FIGURE 3   Liver scan posterior-anterior (A) and lateral (B) showing presence and location of a large lesion in the superior and posterior aspects of the right lobe as indicated by the arrows.

diaphragm and the urgent nature of the case which did not permit delays or multiple procedures. Under these circumstances, the liver was approached intraperitoneally, the abscess located by palpation and needle aspiration. With the needle in place, drainage was accomplished by cautery incision along the needle position into the abscess cavity which often was located in the liver tissues for a distance of 3 to 5 or more cm. To minimize contamination, the operative area and wound edges were walled off by laparotomy sponges before the abscess was opened, and the purulent contents quickly removed by the aspirating tip attached to suction. A large caliber soft rubber tube or Foley catheter was then inserted into the abscess cavity to minimize continuing intraperitoneal contamination and infection,

and it was brought out through a flank stab wound. Soft rubber tissue drains, brought out through a subcostal flank stab wound, were inserted into the subphrenic, in trahepatic, right renal, and right paracolic spaces. The surgical working incision was then closed both in layers and with retention sutures.

Antibiotic Therapy Antibacterial therapy was used in all cases preoperatively, intraoperatively, and postoperatively as indicated. When possible the selection of the antibacterial agent or agents was made preoperatively on the basis of cultures and sensitivity tests made usually on microorganisms isolated from the blood stream. When such cultures were not available preoperatively, the selection of the antibiotic agents was made on the basis of a presumptive etiology until specific information was provided by examination of gram-stained preparations of the pus at the time of operation or later by the results of the cultures and sensitivity tests.

The antimicrobial therapy was continued for variable periods depending upon the size of the abscess, the association of septicemia, and other smaller abscesses, and the patient's postoperative course. In most instances the duration of therapy exceeded 14 days, and occasionally was extended for as long as 10 weeks.

The development of secondary postoperative abscesses was not significant, and the preoperative, operative, and postoperative antibiotic therapy was interpreted as having been helpful in this regard also.

Mortality Mortality in these patients with suppurative disease of the liver was strikingly related to accurate diagnosis and effective drainage. (Table VIII) Unrecognized hepatic abscesses were invariably fatal. In contrast, all patients but one whose liver abscesses were drained survived during the 16-year period. It is interesting to note that this patient died of a massive pulmonary embolism in his postoperative period during which he was recovering from his infection.

In the first two periods of the study a positive diagnosis was made prior to death in only 20 percent and 18 percent of the cases respectively. In the last six-year period, however,

TABLE VII
COMPLICATIONS OF LIVER ABSCESSES
(Group I)

COMPLICATION		No.
Septicemia		17
Rupture into the Right Subphrenic Space		6
Without Other Complications	4	
Without Associated Empyema	4	
With Empyema and Bronchial Communication	1	
Perforation with Generalized Peritonitis		2
Empyema Without Involvement of Subphrenic Space		2
Recurrence of Abscess		1
Obstruction of Hepatic Duct (Intrahepatic)		2
Leakage of Cysts (Preoperative)		1
Pulmonary Embolism (Postoperative)		1

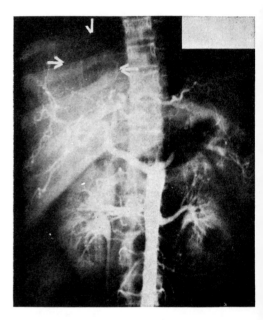

FIGURE 4   Arteriogram including the celiac axis confirming the presence and location of an avascular area in the superior portion of the right lobe of the liver. Convexity of the curved branches of the hepatic artery confirms the presence of the abscess.

a positive diagnosis was made in 80 percent of the cases. This increase in the number of abscesses recognized has permitted a marked reduction in mortality from 80 percent and 82 percent in the first two five-year periods, to 20 percent in the last six years. There has been no mortality in the last nine cases seen by the authors.

The diagnosis of liver abscess has been very difficult until the recent introduction of liver scan techniques using radioisotopes. Between 1955 and 1965 a correct antemortem diagnosis was made in only 19 percent of the cases, and all of the remaining 81 percent were diagnosed at autopsy. By marked contrast, a correct diagnosis was made during the past six years in 80 percent of the cases. This difference was attributable directly to the definitive localizing results of the liver scans and the earlier and more effective operations to drain the abscesses. With the mortality of undrained abscesses being 100 percent during this 16 year study, the significance of early and correct diagnosis has become obvious.

Discussion

Hepatic abscess has been a life-threatening clinical entity of infrequent occurrence. It has consisted of three general types: bacterial or pyogenic, parasitic, and mycotic. In our series of 68 cases, the pyogenic type was by far the most frequently encountered, consisting of two general varieties: (1) a solitary or confluent abscess usually limited to one hepatic lobe and amenable to surgical drainage, and (2) multiple small abscesses throughout both lobes and not amenable to surgical drainage. Our study of 68 patients with liver abscesses seen at the University of Cincinnati Medical Center has given us a better understanding of the nature of this disease and improved methods of diagnosis and treatment.

The observations of others that liver abscess has been a secondary disease with a primary focus usually being demonstrable[1,9,18,19] have been confirmed by our observations. In approximately one-fourth of our cases, however, the primary source was not detectable, and these were classified as cryptogenic. Similar observations have been made by others.[9,18]

TABLE VIII
LIVER ABSCES:: RELATIONSHIP OF DIAGNOSIS,
SURGICAL DRAINAGE, AND MORTALITY
(68 Patients)

Time Period	No. of Cases	Number/% Diagnosed	Number Drained	Mortality in Drained Cases	Mortality No Drainage	Overall Mortality
1955-59	10	2/20%	2	0%	100%	80%
1960-64	11	2/18%	2	0%	100%	82%
1965-70	20	16/80%	16*	6%+	100%	20%

*One abscess decompressed after spontaneous rupture.
*One patient died with a pulmonary embolism in the postoperative period.

The evidence has indicated that the pathways of infection to the liver in our series included direct extension from contiguous disease, the portal vein, the biliary ductal system, the hepatic artery, and the umbilical veins in the newborn infant.

Its incidence as a solitary or confluent lesion has remained relatively constant during the past 16 years. There has been a progressive decrease in the number of cases recognized to have multiple small abscesses of the liver. However, this most likely has been the result of effective antibiotic therapy of the primary non-hepatic disease and its complicating sepsis.

The age incidence has shown two patterns. In the Group I patients with localized abscesses, the age incidence has been distributed relatively evenly throughout all decades of life. In the Group II patients with multiple small abscesses, on the other hand, two peaks of greatest incidence in the extremes of life were noted: the newborn infant and sixth and seventh decades. The similarity of these observations to those observed by us in patients with gram-negative septicemia was of interest.

In the pyogenic abscesses, a variety of aerobic bacteria were cultured from the abscesses in the majority of instances. The aerobic gram-negative bacilli identified included *E. coli, Aerobacter aerogenes, Alkaligenes faecalis, E. intermedia,* and in that order of frequency. Other aerobic bacteria found were the non-hemolytic streptococcus and beta hemolytic streptococcus. During the past

three years, eight of 12 abscesses yielded only anaerobic bacteria, these being anaerobic *Streptococcus sp., Bacteroides,* and *Actinomyces.* Similar observations have also been made by St. John et al [20] and Block et al.[21]

The onset of abscess of the liver has been insidious, its presence obscure, and its localization difficult. The signs and symptoms noted in our patients generally coincided with those described by other authors.[1,6,22,23] While many patients had dull pain and tenderness in the right upper quadrant few had signs which were little more than suggestive of liver abscess. Roentgenograms of the chest and abdomen likewise gave suggestive evidence in some cases, but were of little help in the differential diagnosis. Oral and intravenous cholangiograms were essentially useless as indications of this form of hepatic infection.

In contrast, liver scanning procedures used during the past six years were of great value in indicating preoperatively the presence of hepatic abscesses and their localization. On the basis of this experience, it has been concluded that radio-isotopic scans should be considered in all patients with obscure signs of sepsis.

Selective arteriograms of the celiac axis and hepatic artery have been of more limited value. Their usefulness has been in demonstrating larger avascular areas and confirming defects noted on the liver scans.

The laboratory data of particular diagnostic importance were leucocytosis with a shift to the left, mild anemia, increased alkaline phosphatase levels, decreased serum albumin levels, and increased bromsulphalein retention.

Summary

The experience in a series of 68 patients with liver abscesses seen at the University of Cincinnati Medical Center has been studied to obtain a better understanding of the incidence, etiology, pathogenesis, diagnostic problems, effectiveness of therapy, morbidity, and mortality of this serious disease.

This study has emphasized the fact that the mortality of this life-threatening disease was 100 percent when undiagnosed and undrained surgically. In contrast, there was no mortality in all of the cases but one in which a diagnosis had been made and surgical drainage was instituted.

During the past six years, our capability of diagnosing and localizing abscesses 2 cm or larger has been greatly increased by the use of radio-isotopic liver scanning techniques, aided more recently by hepatic arteriography. The benefits of these new techniques have been obvious in a disease in which the mortality otherwise has been 100 percent when surgical drainage has not been instituted. The more definitive and earlier diagnosis of liver abscesses has permitted life saving surgical drainage with no mortality under the planned and safer conditions thus made possible. In addition, the number of correctly diagnosed cases which could be operated upon successfully was increased.

REFERENCES

1. Ochsner A, DeBakey M and Murray S. Pyogenic abscess of the liver. II. An analysis of forty-seven cases with review of the literature. Am J Surg 40:292-319, 1938.
2. Eliason EL: Phylephlebitis and liver abscess following appendicitis. Surg Gynec & Obst 42: 510-522, 1926.
3. McFadzean JS, Chang KPS and Wong CC: Solitary pyogenic abscess of the liver treated by closed aspiration and antibiotics. A report of 14 consecutive cases with recovery. Brit J Surg 41: 141-152, 1953.
4. Cronin K: Pyogenic abscess of the liver. Gut 2:53-59, 1953.
5. Rayes AI and Reyes DA: Hepatic abscess. An analysis of 86 cases. Int Surg 52:1173-1178, 1969.
6. Ostermiller W and Carter R: Hepatic abscess: Current concepts in diagnosis and management. Arch Surg 94:353-356, 1967.
7. Berke J and Pecora C: Diagnostic problems of pyogenic hepatic abscess. Am J Surg 111:678-682, 1966.
8. Warren KW and Hardy KJ: Pyogenic hepatic abscess. Arch Surg 97:40-45, 1968.
9. Gaisford WD and Mark JBD: Surgical management of hepatic abscess. Am J Surg 118:317-326, 1969.
10. Schuman BM, Block MA, Eyler WR, et al: Liver abscess: Rose Bengal I-131 hepatic photoscan in diagnosis and management. JAMA 187:708-711 1964.
11. Gollin FF, Sims JL and Cameron JR: Liver scanning and liver function tests—a comparative study. JAMA 187:111-116, 1964.
12. Shingleton WW, Taylor LA and Pircher FJ: Radioisotope photoscan of liver in differential diagnosis of upper abdominal disease: Review of 232 cases. Ann Surg 163:685-691, 1966.
13. Gottschalk A: Liver scanning. JAMA 200:630-633, 1967.
14. McCarthy CF, Read AEA, Ross FGM, et al: Ultrasonic scanning of the liver. Quart J Med 36:517-524, 1967.
15. Sparberg M, Gottschalk A and Kirsner JB: Liver abscess complicating regional enteritis: Report of two cases. Gastroenterology 49:548-551, 1965.
16. Holt JM and Sory CJF: Solitary pyogenic liver abscess in patients with diabetes mellitus. Lancet 2:198-200, 1966.
17. Altemeier WA, Todd JC and Inge WW: Gram-negative septicemia: A growing threat. Ann Surg 166:228-240, 1967.
18. Rambo WM and Black HC: Intrahepatic abscess. Am Surg 35:144-148. 1969.
19. Sherman JD and Robbins SL: Changing trends in the casuistics of hepatic abscess. Am J Med 28:943-950, 1960.
20. St. John FB, Pulaski EJ and Ferrer JM: Primary abscess of the liver due to anaerobic nonhemolytic streptococcus. Ann Surg 116:217-222, 1942.
21. Block MA, Schuman BM, Eyler WR, et al: Surgery of liver abscesses. Arch Surg 88:602-610, 1964.

INCREASING INCIDENCE OF FUNGAL INFECTIONS

• Nosocomial factors predispose hospital patients to infections with fungi which under normal conditions do not usually cause infection in man. The clinician and the clinical laboratory must be alert to the possible occurrences of these infections.

EILEEN L. RANDALL, PH.D.

An ever increasing number of fungal infections are being reported, especially those due to opportunistic fungi[1,3]. The reasons for this increased incidence are probably multiple, and some of these are listed in Table 1.

The use of broad-spectrum antibiotics which affect normal flora, especially that of the gastrointestinal tract, is felt to play an important role in the emergence of many fungi, particularly yeast[4,5]

The administration of antimetabolites to patients with malignancies constitutes another important predisposing condition which enables fungi to invade tissue. The deleterious effect of these agents on the mucous membranes of the body, including those of the intestinal tract, provides a ready portal of entry for fungi that are normally found in the gut, such as *Candida albicans*, other *Candida* species, *Torulopsis*, *Trichosporon*, and *Rhodotorula*. The drug-induced granulocytopenia is an important factor in the decreased defense to all types of infections, including those due to fungi.

Corticosteroids have been incriminated as a predisposing factor in the occurrence of fungal infections, especially those due to *Aspergillus*.[5] These agents are known to produce a defective function of the polymorphonuclear leukocyte.

The increased use of immunosuppressive agents, through their effect on the humoral and cellular immunity, constitutes another well known predisposing factor in the occurrence of fungal infections, particularly those caused by *Candida* and *Aspergillus*. As the number of patients undergoing various transplantations increase, we can be certain that there will be observed a concomitant increase in the number of fungal infections.

Urinary bladder instrumentation and the prolonged use of urinary catheters, especially in the female, promote the growth of fungi such as yeast.

The increasingly common use of central venous pressure catheters and indwelling venous catheters for the administration of various fluids constitutes another very important factor in the rising incidence of fungemia.[6]

Patients with tracheostomies commonly become infected with bacteria, and this site can be an important portal of entry into the body of fungi such as yeast.

Certain disease states are associated with a variety of fungal infections and are listed in Table 2. *Mucor* and *Candida* occur in patients with diabetes mellitus. *Aspergillus* fungus balls, aspergillomas, are being seen with increasing frequency in patients with sarcoidosis, particularly those patients with cavitary disease who are receiving steroids. Aspergillomas are being observed also in patients with cavitary disease due to tuberculosis and malignancy. An increased incidence of nocardiosis is seen in patients with alveolar proteino-

Dr. Randall is Microbiologist, Thomas Jefferson University Hospital; Associate Professor of Microbiology; Associate Professor of Pathology, Jefferson Medical College.

TABLE 1

SOME CAUSES FOR THE INCREASED INCIDENCE OF FUNGAL INFECTIONS

1. Use of Broad-Spectrum Antibiotics
2. Administration of Antimetabolites
3. Administration of Corticosteroids
4. Administration of Immunosuppressive Agents
5. Use of Indwelling Intravenous Catheters
6. Use of Urinary Tract Catheters
7. Tracheostomy

---

sis. It is a well established fact that patients with Hodgkin's disease, leukemia, and other blood dyscrasias are more prone to fungal infections caused by *Cryptococcus, Candida,* and *Aspergillus.* The burned patient is quite susceptible to fungal infections, and *Mucor* and *Candida* are often incriminated. Lastly, patients who have undergone surgical procedures appear to be more prone to fungal infections.[5] The occurrence of *Candida* endocarditis in patients whose heart valves have been replaced is not uncommon, and the finding of *Aspergillus* in the heart muscle of patients who have undergone heart transplantation has been reported.

At Thomas Jefferson University Hospital during the past several years we have seen an actual increase in the number of patients with fungal infections. A greater number of specimens are being sent to the laboratory requesting fungal cultures than were sent even two years ago, and a greater number of fungal isolates are being made.

In Table 3 can be seen the numbers of "mold" isolations that have been made during two separate two-year periods, 1967-1968 and 1969-1970. The most common mold isolated is *Aspergillus,* and this is often a laboratory contaminant. It is often difficult for the laboratory to attach clinical significance to the mere isolation of *Aspergillus* from clinical specimens because of the ubiquitous nature of this organism. The diagnosis of aspergillosis, therefore, is usually made on clinical evidence plus the repeated isolation of the organism from the patient. The number of isolations of *Aspergillus* during the last two-year period

have decreased from 529-470 — a reflection of less contamination in the laboratory. *Penicillium* is the next most common mold isolation and has been considered contamination with the exception of one case where *Penicillium* was isolated from a lung abscess of a patient from whom *Coccidioides* was also isolated. It was felt that the *Penicillium* was a secondary invader. Relatively few isolations of other molds are made. Mold isolations over this four-year period represent 27 per cent of the total fungal isolates.

Table 4 shows the number of "yeast" isolations that have been made during these same two-year periods. The single most common isolate is *Candida albicans,* and the number of isolates doubled during the last two-year period, going from 761 to 1534. The number of *Candida* species not *C. albicans* went from 311 to 619 and the isolation of *Geotrichum* from 30 to 120. The numbers of *Torulopsis* and *Trichosporon* isolates also showed increases during this period. It can be seen from comparing Tables 3 and 4 that yeast isolates are most commonly made, and they represent 73 per cent of the total fungal isolates.

Yeast are not only the most commonly isolated fungi, but they also constitute the majority of the clinically significant isolates. In Table 5 can be seen the numbers of patients from whom yeast have been isolated from blood. The number of patients are divided into three separate five-year periods. Again *Candida albicans* has been the most common species, and there has been a sharp increase in the number of infected patients during the

TABLE 2

DISEASE STATES WHICH ARE ASSOCIATED WITH FUNGAL INFECTIONS

1. Diabetes Mellitus
2. Sarcoid
3. Tuberculosis
4. Malignancy
5. Alveolar Proteinosis
6. Hodgkin's, Leukemia, and Other Blood Dyscrasias
7. Burned Patients
8. Patients with Surgical Procedures

	1967 - 1968	1969 - 1970	TOTAL
Aspergillus	529	470	999
Penicillium	52	53	105
Unidentified Mold	26	8	34
Cladosporium	13	11	24
Paecilomyces	6	14	20
Rhizopus	4	15	19
Other Molds	47	66	113
Total	677	637	1314

Molds — 27% of Total Fungal Isolates

TABLE 3

MOLD ISOLATIONS

Thomas Jefferson
University Hospital

last five-year period rising from 7 in 1961-1965 to 41 during the 1966-1970 period. *Candida* species not *albicans* is the next most commonly isolated, and it too has shown a sharp increase during the last five-year period going from 1 to 3 to 30. Unidentified yeast are those that were discarded or died before proper identification was made. The number of patients from whom *Cryptococcus* has been isolated have not increased during these periods. Three patients with *Torulopsis* and one patient with *Geotrichum* have been seen during the last five-year period. During 1970 twenty-one patients had fungemia due to various species of yeast, and a common isolate was *Candida parapsilosis*. Many of these patients had indwelling venous catheters.

Yeast are most commonly recovered from blood cultures when pour plates of the patient's blood are made. Many strains of *Candida* will not grow in commercially available broth bottles, presumably because of fungistatic or fungicidal substances normally present in blood. Colonies of yeast in pour plates can be detected as early as eighteen hours after the blood culture is taken.

Table 6 shows the numbers of patients with systemic fungal infections seen during the last fifteen years. These represent all types of infections, including pneumonic processes, aspergillomas, fungemias, central nervous system disease, and other systemic organ involvement. Again they are divided into three five-year periods, and a definite increase in the total numbers is seen during the last five-year period: 57 from 1956-1960, 56 from 1961-1965 and 155 from 1966-1970. *Candida* species was

the etiologic agent in 122 patients (46 per cent) and *Aspergillus* in 71 patients (25 per cent). The 27 patients with unidentified mold were patients in whom a diagnosis of fungal infection was made at the time of post mortem, and the organism was not identified as to genus. Most of these were probably due to *Candida* or *Aspergillus*.

Infections due to cryptococci have remained at almost the same level throughout the 15-year period.

The numbers of patients infected with *Nocardia* and *Actinomyces* do not represent the total number of patients with infections due to these organisms. This table represents those that were found to be cultured positive in the mycology division, and most of these infections are diagnosed in the bacteriology division.

The patients with *Torulopsis, Mucor, Coccidioides, Histoplasma,* and *Geotrichum* were so few in number that evaluations as to their increasing appearance cannot be made.

Laboratory diagnosis of systemic fungal infections is at times difficult. The mere isolation of certain fungi such as yeast and *Aspergillus* is not proof of infection as these organisms, especially yeast, are many times part of the normal flora of the body. *Aspergillus* is a common airborne contaminant of our environment, and isolation of it from culture media commonly occurs.

When *Candida* has invaded tissue, the organism appears in its hyphal form. Thus, if smears are made from urine, areas of thrush,

135

	1967 - 1968	1969 - 1970	TOTAL
Candida Albicans	761	1534	2295
Candida Species	311	619	930
Geotrichum	30	120	150
Torulopsis	42	62	104
Trichosporon	22	44	66
Other Yeast	27	26	53
Total	1193	2405	3598

Yeast — 73% of Total Fungal Isolates

TABLE 4

YEAST ISOLATIONS

Thomas Jefferson
University Hospital

or feces, and yeast forms with pseudohyphae are seen, tissue invasion should be suspected. The interpretation of a patient's sputa showing yeast forms with pseudohyphae is more difficult as the lung might not be involved, but the yeast may be present in another portion of the respiratory tree. Sputa obtained by transtracheal aspiration would be more easily evaluated.

Torulopsis is beginning to be reported as a cause of opportunistic infections. It has been increasingly seen at our hospital especially from the urinary tract and has been isolated from blood cultures of three patients. This organism should be suspected from patients when small yeast about half the size of *Candida* that do not form hyphae are observed on gram-stained smears or wet mounts. At times *Torulopsis* does not grow well on blood agar and only pinpoint colonies will be observed. It grows well on Sabourauds's dextrose agar.

Geotrichum is suspected when rectangular yeast cells are seen in gram-stained smears. It should be differentiated from a closely related genus, *Trichosporon*, which culturally mimics *Geotrichum*. Both of these organisms are part of normal bowel flora and are being observed as causes of fungal infections.

India ink stains of spinal fluid or other body fluids enable the capsule of *Cryptococcus* to be observed. Periodic acid shift stains, such as Gridley's, stain the polysaccharide capsule well in tissue slides containing cryptococci. When cryptococcosis is suspected and the organism is not observed in spinal fluid, large amounts of urine, including that obtained at the very end of urination, should be centrifuged and cultured. *Cryptococcus neoformans* is being isolated from sputa from patients without evidence of clinical disease. Perhaps this organism can be found as part of normal flora.

Histoplasma, best observed in Wright or Giemsa stained preparation of clinical specimens, is being observed in patients with Hodgkin's disease or other blood dyscrasias. The organism at times is difficult to isolate in culture from sputa, especially if *Pseudomonas* is also present. In tissue sections when few organisms are present, they can be detected easily with a silver methenamine stain. The very small size, two to four micra, of these organisms makes identification fairly easy.

Actinomycosis does not appear to be increasing in frequency. *Actinomyces* is an endogenous organism, and the disease usually occurs after trauma to the mouth area or following abdominal surgery. The organism must be differentiated from *Nocardia* in original smears as both are branching gram-positive rods. *Nocardia* is usually acid fast, especially when stained in smears of specimens containing protein material. In tissue *Actinomyces* grows in colonies referred to as sulfur granules, and *Nocardia* does not. Both elicit a polymorphonuclear response in tissue. *Actinomyces* in tissue must be differentiated from organisms causing botryomycosis, a bacterial disease. In certain patients staphylococci, *Pseudomonas*, and other organisms will grow as granules and, in H and E tissue sections, these are indistinguishable from those produced by *Actinomyces*. A gram-stained preparation of the section will provide the diagnosis.

	1956 - 1960	1961 - 1965	1966 - 1970	TOTAL
Candida Albicans	0	7	41	48
Candida Species	1	3	30	34
Unidentified Yeast	2	3	6	11
Cryptococcus	3	0	1	4
Torulopsis	0	0	3	3
Geotrichum	0	0	1	1
Total	6	13	82	101

TABLE 5

YEAST - BLOOD CULTURES

Thomas Jefferson
University Hospital

Nocardiosis does appear to be increasing in frequency. It is not uncommon in patients with carcinomatosis of the lung. We have observed one patient undergoing hemodialysis whose A-V shunt area became infected with *Nocardia*.

Zygomycosis or phycomycosis caused by *Mucor* and *Rhizopus* species has not been observed often by us. However, during the last several months three patients at post mortem were shown to have systemic disease due to these organisms. On tissue section zygomycosis can be differentiated easily from aspergillosis. *Mucor* and related organisms are nonseptate, have a wider diameter than *Aspergillus*, and branch at right angles. They appear ribbon-like in tissue. *Aspergillus* has septate hyphae and branch at more acute angles.

Aspergillosis is commonly diagnosed at our medical center, and an increasing number of patients are becoming infected each year. Many of these present as aspergillomas superimposed on cavitary disease due to sarcoid, tuberculosis, or malignancy. Some of these spread to invade the parenchyma of the lung, and some remain localized in the cavity as fungus balls. Other patients, especially those receiving antimetabolites or steroids, or both, are not diagnosed until post mortem examination. Systemic spread of the organism in these patients is at times observed, but usually the lesions are confined to the parenchyma of the lung.

In Table 7, thirty patients in whom a diagnosis of aspergillosis has been made are listed with their underlying disease and whether or not the radiology and precipitin test were positive. All of the patients except two showed

	1956 - 1960	1961 - 1965	1966 - 1970	TOTAL
Candida	22	23	77	122
Aspergillus	13	8	50	71
Unidentified Mold	15	12	0	27
Cryptococcus	4	5	5	14
Unidentified Yeast	1	4	4	9
Nocardia	2	1	6	9
Actinomyces	0	2	5	7
Torulopsis	0	0	3	3
Mucor	0	1	1	2
Coccidioides	0	0	2	2
Histoplasma	0	0	1	1
Geotrichum	0	0	1	1
Total	57	56	155	268

TABLE 6

SYSTEMIC FUNGAL INFECTIONS

Thomas Jefferson
University Hospital

Underlying Disease		Radiology		Serology	
Sarcoidosis	19	Positive	18	Positive	12
				Not Done	5
				Negative	2
Post Cyst	3	Positive	3	Positive	2
				Not Done	1
Tuberculosis	6	Postitive	6	Positive	6
Alveolar Proteinosis	1	Positive	1	Positive	1
Allergic Aspergillosis	1	Negative	1	Positive	1

TABLE 7

ASPERGILLOSIS

Thomas Jefferson
University Hospital

roentgenologic evidence of disease. Of these two, one had sarcoidosis and one allergic aspergillosis. All of the patients tested except two with sarcoidosis showed a positive precipitin test against antigens prepared from various strains of *Aspergillus*.

The diagnosis of aspergilloma is confirmed by roentgenologic evidence, recovery of the organisms from culture, and serologic studies. When these aspergillomas are surgically removed, wet mount of the contents will reveal either masses of septate hyphae or, in some cases, conidiophores and spores. The finding of spores must depend upon how well the cavities are aerated. Some patients with aspergillomas will cough up portions of the ball, and microscopic examination will slow the organism.

Sputa from some patients with *Aspergillus* present in the parenchyma of the lungs and from many of those with aspergillomas will show branching septate hyphae on wet mount along with numerous polymorphonuclear white cells. Gram-stained preparations are practically worthless as aspergilli do not stain well with this stain, and only a very small amount of sputum is examined.

Summary

A marked increase in the number of patients with fungal infections has been observed over the last five-year period compared to the previous ten years. The two most common organisms isolated from the infected patients are *Candida* and *Aspergillus* species. Two disease processes most commonly seen during the last two-year period are aspergillomas superimposed on sarcoidosis and tuberculosis and fungemia due to *Candida* species. It is postulated that even more fungal infections will be observed in the future because those patients more susceptible to these opportunistic organisms are commonly seen in our medical centers today.

ACKNOWLEDGEMENT

The author wishes to thank Irving Abrahams, Ph.D., Director of Laboratories and Research, Meadowbrook Hospital, Plainview, N.Y. for his kind performance of the precipitin tests for aspergillosis.

REFERENCES

1. Utz JP: The spectrum of opportunistic fungus infections. Lab Invest 11:1018-1025, 1962.
2. Louria DB: Treatment of opportunistic fungal infections. Mod Treat 3:1099-1106, 1966.
3. Marks MI, Langston C and Eickhoff TC: *Torulopsis Glabrata* —an opportunistic pathogen in man. NEJM 283:1131-1135, 1970.
4. Seelig MS: Mechanisms by which antibiotics increase the evidence and severity of candidiasis and alter the immunological defense. Bact Rev 30:442-459, 1966.
5. Louria DB: Deep-seated mycotic infections, allergy to fungi and mycotoxins. NEJM 277:1065-1071, 1126-1134, 1967.
6. Rodrigues RJ, Chinya H, Wolff WI, et al: *Torulopsis Glabrata* fungemia during prolonged intravenous alimentation therapy. NEJM 284:540-541, 1971.

FEVER OF UNKNOWN ETIOLOGY

- A persistent methodical approach to the history and physical examination in the patient with fever of undetermined origin will frequently lead to the reward of uncovering the proper diagnosis.

DONALD B. LOURIA, M.D.

The first crude clinical thermometer was developed by Sanctorius in the early 1600's. Almost 100 years later, Gabriel Fahrenheit provided the medical profession with the instrument needed to follow accurately the temperature patterns in various disease states. Since that time, a great many astute clinicians have made shrewd diagnoses based, in large part, on the fever curves in the front of every patient's hospital chart. Perhaps no diagnostic challenge fascinates the diagnostician as much as the fever of unknown origin (FUO). Alt and Barker[1] of the Peter Bent Brigham Hospital collected 101 such cases in 1930, and Hamman and Wainright[2] summarized 90 cases with high fever in 1936. In the former series, 57 were febrile for over ten days; a final diagnosis was made in 23 of these cases, the most frequently diagnosed diseases being rheumatic fever (6), tuberculosis (6), and carcinoma (3). In the Hamman and Wainright series, 44 cases were solved, the most frequent diagnoses being syphilis (10), tuberculosis (9), hypernephroma (5), Hodgkin's disease (4), brucellosis (4), hidden abscesses (3), and carcinoma (2).

Chester Keefer, a masterful clinician, collected 80 solved cases in a delightful, brief monograph published in 1955 and entitled "Prolonged and Perplexing Fever."[3] Of the 80 cases, the fever in 51 instances was due to specific infectious agents, including eight due

to the tubercle bacillus, six due to species of brucella, and two caused by salmonella species. Additionally, there were four cases of bacterial endocarditis, ten tumors, and four cases of lymphoma. In three instances the fever was due to hepatic cirrhosis, and in two other cases the final diagnosis was thyrotoxicosis.

In the last 30 years, we have added little clinically to the FUO entity. Indeed, I recently referred to my 1952 medical school lecture on FUO delivered by Dr. Louis Weinstein, Professor of Medicine at Boston's Tufts Medical School, and, by general agreement, the most adroit American physician in correctly diagnosing fevers of undetermined origin. With a few small additions, that lecture would be as applicable now as it was about 20 years ago.

Petersdorf and Beeson emphasize this point in a comprehensive article in 1961, and the former in a brief review in 1969.[4,5] They noted that of those with unexplained fever, 40 per cent will have a specific infection, 20 per cent will be found to suffer from tumors, and 20 per cent from collagen vascular disease. In another 10 per cent, the diagnoses will include pulmonary emboli, drug fever, sarcoid and malingering.

Summarized in Table 1 are some of the more frequent and some of the less frequent causes of FUO.

In the last decade, our knowledge about the FUO has been enhanced by the following observations:

Dr. Louria is Professor and Chairman, Department of Public Health and Preventive Medicine, College of Medicine and Dentistry of New Jersey at Newark.

TABLE 1

THIRTY CAUSES OF FEVER OF UNDETERMINED ORIGIN

FREQUENT	LESS FREQUENT	INFREQUENT
Tuberculosis	Hypernephroma	Regional enteritis
Polyarteritis	Other tumors	Ulcerative colitis
Lymphoma	Endocarditis	Sarcoid
Drugs	Malingering	Thyrotoxicosis
	Hidden abscess	Cirrhosis or fatty liver
	Pylephlebitis	Periodic fever
	Osteomyelitis	Adrenal tumor
	Pyelonephritis	Thyroiditis
	Diverticulitis	Congestive failure
	Salmonellosis	Hyperlipemia
	Malaria	Hypothalamic lesions
	Pulmonary emboli	Brucellosis
	Cytomegalic inclusion virus	
	Cholangitis	

(1) Cytomegalic inclusion disease virus (CMV) may induce a prolonged fever in an otherwise healthy individual. In a recently published series from Denmark, CMV infection was the presumed diagnosis in six of 34 cases of FUO.[6] A substantial peripheral blood lymphocytosis or monocytosis may be noted, and this in itself should suggest the diagnosis. The severity of illness is extraordinarily variable; the patient may appear toxic or virtually asymptomatic. The duration of fever is also unpredictable, ranging from a few days to several months.

(2) Toxoplasmosis may present as persistent fever. Usually cervical or supraclavicular adenopathy is present, but this is not invariably so; and there may be substantial peripheral lymphocytosis. A toxoplasma dye test and determination of complement fixing antibody titers should be of great help in establishing the diagnosis.

(3) Although sarcoid may be manifested as an FUO, this is quite infrequent; more often fever is not a significant part of the clinical picture of sarcoidosis.

(4) Patients suffering from underlying reticuloendothelial system malignancy, especially those being treated with immunosuppressive agents and/or adrenal corticosteroids, are inordinately susceptible to superinfection due to *Pneumocystis carinii*, CMV, *Candida sp.*, *Aspergillus sp.*, or gram-negative enteric bacteria. Such infections may present as an FUO. These organisms also cause clinical disease in patients who have undergone kidney or heart transplantations and are being treated with immunosuppressive drugs.[7-8]

(5) Personnel returning from duty in Southeast Asia may have fever due to dengue, the virus of chickungunya fever, scrub typhus, leptospirosis, or melioidosis.[9] Furthermore, the patient may have left the endemic area some time ago; in the case of scrub typhus, eg, the incubation period may be as long as 21 days.

(6) Malaria must be considered in virtually every case of unexplained fever in young persons or travelers. An epidemic, initiated by a returning Vietnam veteran, has recently been documented in California among young persons taking heroin intravenously.[10] Even if one takes prophylactic anti-malaria drugs conscientiously while in the endemic area, malaria can become apparent after leaving the endemic area, but more often, the prophylactic regimen has not been followed. Although the incubation period for *P. falciparum, P.*

ovale, and *P. malariae* is less than one month, there may be a hiatus of several months between infection and clinical signs in *P. vivax* infections.[11] Consequently, the patient may be far removed from the area in which infection took place. *P. falciparum* infections can relapse up to 18 months later, *P. vivax* and *P. ovale* up to three years later, and *P. malariae* for five to fifty years after initiation of infection.[11]

(7) In children, unusual cases for FUO are familial dysautonomia, viralizing adrenal hyperplasia, hyperthyroidism, and infantile cortical hyperostosis.[12]

(8) Certain signs should suggest specific diagnoses:

      (a) fundal infiltrates — tuberculosis or collagen disease. Careful fundoscopic examination should be performed every few days on every patient with an FUO, dilating the pupils, if necessary.

      (b) red, weeping eyes — polyarteritis.[13]

      (c) conjunctivitis — lupus erythematosus, tuberculosis.

      (d) trapezius soreness — subdiaphragmatic abscess.[13]

      (e) sternal tenderness — marrow invasion.[13]

      (f) muscle tenderness — polyarteritis.

      (g) back pain — staphylococcal or salmonella osteomyelitis or enterococcal aortic valve endocarditis.

(9) In the adult, hyperlipemia, temporal arteritis, atrial myxoma, and thyroiditis have all been emphasized as infrequent causes of FUO.

(10) The erythrocyte sedimentation rate should be determined in every case; if it is normal, the prognosis is good, whether or not a specific diagnosis is established.[14] A normal sedimentation rate should also spur further consideration of the possibility the patient is malingering.

The following cases illustrate some of the pitfalls in arriving at a correct diagnosis.

Case 1

A 26-year-old man suffered from disabling arthritis, leaving him unable to turn himself. The administration of adrenal glucocorticoids resulted in mild improvement, but after two months of therapy, he developed unexplained fever. After ten days of fever, a consultation was obtained. Examination revealed little, and questioning of the nurses indicated he had no decubiti. A diagnosis of steroid-induced arteritis was considered seriously, but that day somebody turned the patient over, saw a subcutaneous bulge and drained over 500 ml of frank pus.

Comment: This case illustrates the consequences of not doing the physical examination oneself. Here, the patient could not turn himself, and the physician was contented with the assurance that there were no focal lesions on or under the skin in the buttock area. This obviously makes no sense. If the staff had noted a buttock lesion, they would have attended to it, and there would have been no need for the advice of a consultant. Failure to examine the skin or the teeth (for an apical abscess) will result occasionally in an embarrassing mis-diagnosis.

Case 2

A 24-year-old man was hospitalized because of shaking chills and fever of two weeks' duration. The history contributed little else. Physical examination was negative. Laboratory studies showed a mild elevation of the alkaline phosphatase, and on liver biopsy some polymorphonuclear leukocyte infiltration was evident. Although it then appeared clear that there was hepatic infection, the exact nature of the disease process was unclear. Cultures of blood and liver biopsy showed no growth. At laparotomy, a retrocecal appendix that had ruptured was found. Another history was obtained, focusing on the known diagnosis of appendicitis with rupture and pylephlebitis. The patient then gave a perfectly clear and classic story of mid-abdominal pain that moved to the right lower quadrant. This lasted for eight hours, disappearing after his physician, contacted by 'phone, ordered a cathartic. One week later, the fever and chills started.

Comment: The physicians all concentrated on the nature of the illness from the time the fever began. Vague questions were asked about previous illnesses, but no one thought to ask specifically about appendiceal-type pain in the recent past, and the patient did not volunteer the information. There is just no substitute for taking another detailed and thoughtful history when faced with an FUO. Each of the major diagnostic possibilities listed in Table 1 should be considered, and the history sequentially focused on each possibility.

Case 3

A 42-year-old woman was hospitalized because of fever to 103-104 F each night. History and physical examination were totally unrewarding, and blood cultures were negative. Liver function tests were also normal. Skin tests showed a negative first-strength tuberculin, a moderately positive intermediate strength and a strongly positive second strength PPD. After three weeks of bed rest, she appeared much improved, and the temperature now did not rise above 101 F by rectum. At that time, a liver biopsy was taken and showed caseating granulomas in which typical tubercle bacilli were seen.

Comment: We tend to forget that in disseminated tuberculosis the patient may become virtually afebrile merely on bed rest, and that liver involvement, as in this case, may be prominent even though all liver function tests are normal. In any patient with an unexplained fever and a positive tuberculin test, this diagnosis should be considered foremost.

Case 4

A 79-year-old woman was hospitalized because of weakness, fever, and muscle aches of three weeks' duration. Physical examination on admission showed no abnormalities. Laboratory studies revealed negative blood, urine, and stool cultures. The alkaline phosphatase was minimally elevated. Febrile agglutinins were negative, as was the tuberculin skin test. White blood cell count was normal, and there was no anemia. Her fever persisted, the daily peak almost always being recorded in the morning. At the end of three weeks of hospitalization, consultation was requested. Physical examination was un-

changed except for moderate muscle atrophy unaccompanied by tenderness. A diagnosis of biliary tract obstruction and ascending cholangitis secondary to tumor or stones was made, with an alternative diagnosis of tumor involving the liver. Subsequent cervical node and muscle biopsies showed necrotizing vasculitis (polyarteritis).

Comment: In this case, the diagnosis should have been made immediately on the basis of the temperature pattern. Persistent fever with a morning spike is usually due to tuberculosis, polyarteritis or salmonellosis. The tuberculin skin test was negative, and cultures as well as serological tests did not support a diagnosis of salmonellosis. This left only polyarteritis. I actually made that diagnosis on looking at the temperature chart before seeing the patient, but made two mistakes that led to an incorrect shift in diagnosis. First, I ascribed the moderate muscle atrophy to lying in bed and gave too little emphasis to the initial aches, because at the time of examination, I found no muscle tenderness. Second, I talked myself out of the diagnosis of polyarteritis because of the alkaline phosphatase elevation; but it is well known that polyarteritis can cause marked abnormalities in liver function.[15] Similar attention to the temperature pattern may also be helpful in leishmaniasis and gonococcal endocarditis, which often cause a double temperature spike each day, once in the morning and once in the evening.

Case 5

A 36-year-old woman was hospitalized because of nocturnal fever to 103 F for a period of four weeks. Physical examination was entirely normal. Laboratory studies, erythrocyte sedimentation rate included, were normal except for a mild peripheral eosinophilia of 9 per cent. Cholecystogram, intravenous pyelogram, and long bone x-rays were negative. The fever persisted, and because of a questionable abdominal mass, an exploratory laparotomy was performed. No definite pathology was found, but several vessels were biopsied because the surgeon observed that the vessels felt firm on palpation. All biopsies showed normal tissue. The diagnostic enigma was solved when the patient's husband informed the staff that he thought his wife was heating the thermometer. Careful observations thereafter confirmed that this was so. The mild eosinophilia persisted without explanation.

Comment: The patient underwent many expensive tests and abdominal surgery unnecessarily. The diagnosis should have been suspected when the erythrocyte sedimentation rate was found to be normal. Even feeling the skin when the thermometer read 103 F would have obviated the prolonged hospitalization. The staff was fooled because they attributed too much significance to the eosinophilia, and because they accepted the fever as valid on the grounds that the elevation occurred only during the evening. However, today many sophisticated persons are fully aware of the normal diurnal temperature variation-pattern, and even with a curve that appears due to organic disease, it is still necessary to make sure that the fever is not factitious.

Case 6

A 42-year-old man was hospitalized with a six-month history of intermittent fever of up to 103 F by rectum. He had traveled extensively, and despite an entirely negative physical examination, an amebic liver abscess was suspected. None was found, and an extensive laboratory examination showed only an elevated erythrocyte sedimentation rate and an increased serum alpha$_2$ globulin. For three weeks he remained febrile and undiagnosed. Then the fourth house officer dealing with the case decided to take a completely new history, going through the diagnostic possibilities one by one. When he reached the category of thyroid abnormalities, he asked specifically about transient discomfort on swallowing. The patient remembered a ten-day period at the beginning of his illness, but the discomfort was so mild he had forgotten all about it. Physical examination showed minimal, if any, throat tenderness, but serum PBI, iodine uptake studies and thyroid biopsy all confirmed the diagnosis of subacute thyroiditis.

Comment: This case shows the value of a careful history, taken repeatedly if necessary, focusing on specific diagnostic possibilities.

Case 7*

A 31-year-old man suffered from Gaucher's disease for which he had undergone splenectomy. Because of bone marrow hypoplasia and profound anemia, he was repeatedly given blood transfusions. Several weeks after onset of transfusions, he developed shaking chills and fever to 105 F by rectum. An extensive workup at two hospitals, including stool, blood, and urine cultures, did not provide a diagnosis. The only change in his laboratory examination was an increase in the lymphocyte percentage in his peripheral blood smear from 40 to 63. Over a six-week period, the fever lessened, but he was still febrile to about 102 F on most days, usually in the evening. Because of a positive intermediate strength tuberculin test, he was treated for presumably active tuberculosis, despite a negative chest x-ray. When the fever persisted, treatment for culture negative bacterial endocarditis was instituted; this was justified on the basis of fever and a systolic heart murmur, although it was recognized the murmur could well be due to the substantial anemia. Only after six weeks of fever was proper attention paid to the increased peripheral lymphocyte count. Although urine cultures did not show cytomegalic inclusion virus, complement fixation studies showed a diagnostic increase in antibody against the virus.

Comment: Shaking chills do not exclude the diagnosis of tuberculosis, but they do militate against it. There is a natural inclination to make a presumptive diagnosis of endocarditis in the presence of fever and a murmur, even if blood cultures are negative. But ordinarily, this impulse should be resisted unless there is clear evidence of underlying valvular heart disease or a convincing clinical picture indicating bacterial endocarditis: ie, clubbing, petechiae, emboli to the eye or extremities, Osler's nodes, etc. If the patient has an FUO, the likelihood of endocarditis being present in the absence of positive cultures is directly related to how closely the clinical picture resembles classic bacterial endocarditis. If the diagnosis is based solely on the presence of a murmur of questionable significance, it is likely the

---

* This patient was seen in consultation with Dr. Alvin Rosenberg of Morristown, N.J.

diagnosis is incorrect. In all such patients, blood cultures should be obtained in hypertonic media since these may occasionally be positive when routine cultures are negative. It is well to remember that cytomegalic inclusion virus infection can occur in healthy or compromised hosts, may persist for many weeks, and may be associated with either severe or mild clinical illness; and, of course, this diagnosis should always be suspected strongly in a patient who has recently received blood transfusions.

Case 8*

A 69-year-old woman was hospitalized for anemia and a 24-pound weight loss over a two-month period. Physical examination showed mild splenomegaly, and laboratory study revealed a white blood count of 3000 per mm^3 with a normal differential count. First and second strength tuberculin tests were negative. Liver biopsy revealed a small number of polymorphonuclear leukocytes. Because of these findings, a laparotomy was performed. This showed hepatosplenomegaly, and open liver biopsy again revealed polymorphonuclear leukocytes in modest numbers. Cultures of the liver biopsy were negative. Fever persisted for two more months despite intensive antibiotic therapy, and the spleen increased in size. Innumerable blood cultures were sterile, and a third liver biopsy was interpreted as pericholangitis. Despite additional antimicrobials, the relentless deterioration continued. At autopsy, the spleen and

* This patient was seen in consultation with Dr. Bernard Brill of Brooklyn, N.Y.

liver showed many Reed-Sternberg cells characteristic of Hodgkin's disease.

Comment: This difficult case emphasizes that even multiple negative biopsies do not eliminate the possibility of an infiltrating lymphoma. In this case, splenectomy was attempted at the time of laparotomy, but this attempt had to be abandoned because of hypotension. In retrospect, the clue was the white blood cell count. In ascending cholangitis or pylephlebitis, it is rarely this low. Modest leukopenia and moderate splenomegaly in an older person is lymphoma or tuberculosis until proved otherwise.

REFERENCES

1. Alt HL and Barker MH: Fever of unknown origin. JAMA 94: 1457-1460, 1930.
2. Hamman L and Wainwright CW: The diagnosis of obscure fever. The diagnosis of unexplained high fever. Bull Johns Hopkins Hosp 58:307-331, 1936.
3. Keefer CS and Leard SE: Prolonged and Perplexing Fevers. Boston, Little, Brown and Co, 1955.
4. Petersdorf RG and Beeson PB: Fever of unknown origin, report of 100 cases. Medicine 40:1-30, 1961.
5. Petersdorf RG: Fever of unknown origin. Ann Intern Med 70:864-866, 1969.
6. Effersoe P: Fever of unknown origin. A follow-up study of 34 patients discharged without diagnosis. Danish Med Bull 15:240-244, 1968.
7. Stinson EB, Biber CP, Griepp RB, et al: Infectious complications following cardiac transplantation in man. Ann Intern Med 74:1-12, 1971.
8. Rifkind D, Marchioro TL, Schneck SA, et al: Systemic fungal infection complicating renal transplantation and immunosuppressive therapy. Amer J Med 43:28-38, 1967.
9. Gilbert DN, Moore Jr, WL, Hedberg CL, et al: Potential medical problems in personnel returning from Vietnam. Ann Intern Med 68:662-678, 1968.
10. Kearns OA, Huntington RW, Roberto RR, et al: Epidemiologic Notes and Reports. Induced malaria — California. Morbidity and Mortality 20 (#12) March 27, 1971.
11. Bruce-Chwatt LJ: Malaria epidemiology. Brit Med J 2:91-93, 1971.
12. Cone Jr, TE: Diagnosis and treatment: Children with fevers. Pediatrics 43:290-293, 1969.
13. Tumulty PA: Topics in Clinical Medicine. The patient with fever of undetermined origin. A diagnostic challenge. Johns Hopkins Med J 120:95-106, 1967.
14. Bottiger LE: Fever of unknown origin. Acta Medica Scan 147:133-148, 1954.
15. Mowrey FH and Lundberg EA: The clinical manifestations of essential polyangiitis (periarteritis nodosa) with emphasis on the hepatic manifestations. Ann Intern Med 40:1145-1164, 1954.

DIFFERENTIATION OF UPPER FROM LOWER URINARY TRACT INFECTIONS

• The primary physician treating patients with urinary tract infection should be made aware of the importance of determining whether a particular patient is suffering from urinary tract infection localized to the lower tract or if such infection also involves the kidney.

MARVIN TURCK, M.D.

The differentiation of renal from bladder bacteriuria is difficult on clinical grounds alone especially in the asymptomatic patient. Since recognition of renal involvement may be useful not only in defining groups of patients for epidemiologic and therapeutic studies, but also for guiding the duration and intensity of treatment in an individual patient, an accurate laboratory method for localizing the site of urinary tract infection is needed. To date, only bilateral ureteral catheterization has been shown to localize infection with relative certainty.[1,2] However, ureteral catheterization cannot be justified for the routine evaluation of patients with recurrent bacteriuria, and there has been a continued search for less cumbersome methods of localizing infection.

Materials and Methods

One hundred patients, 97 women and three men, with well documented recurrent infections of the urinary tract were subjected to bilateral ureteral catheterizations employing methods previously described from this laboratory.[2] All these patients had previously received several courses of antimicrobial therapy with various agents, but infection had persisted or recurred. Extensive urologic evalu-

ation had not revealed surgically remediable lesions or obstructive uropathy in most patients. However, nine had renal calculi or nephrocalcinosis, and vesicoureteral reflux was found in an additional three women. All but two of the patients had serum creatinine values below 1.5 mg per 100 ml. The majority of patients were asymptomatic at the time of ureteral catheterization, and none had acute clinical pyelonephritis.

The purpose of the present report is to correlate the site of infection with the results of three techniques, 1) serum antibody response, 2) maximal urinary concentrating ability, and 3) urinary beta-glucuronidase activity, which have been employed in our laboratory in an attempt to distinguish between upper and lower urinary tract infection. The methods used for selection of patients and performance of these tests have been described in detail in previous publications from this laboratory.[3-5]

Results

Results of Serum Antibody Response. The results of hemagglutinating antibody titers determined in 79 patients are summarized in Figure 1, which also depicts the species of organism cultured from these patients at the time of bilateral ureteral catheterization. When the antibody titer of serum was compared with the site of infection, most patients with a renal origin for their bacteriuria tended to have a distribution of titers similar to that

Dr. Turck is Associate Professor of Medicine, University of Washington, and Chief of Medicine. United States Public Health Service Hospital, Seattle, Washington.

These studies were supported in part by research grant AI06311 and training grant AI146. National Institutes of Allergy and Infectious Diseases, National Institutes of Health, Bethesda, Md. Part of these studies was supported by a grant (RR-133) from the General Clinical Research Centers Program of the Division of Research Resources, National Institutes of Health.

145

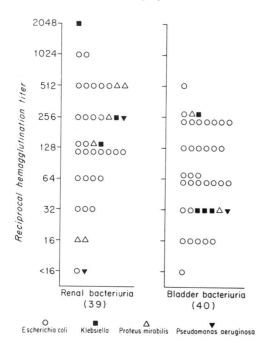

Figure 1

Reciprocal Hemagglutination Titers in Serum in Patients with Bacteriuria. (Reprinted with permission. Ref. 3.)

residual antibody activity after 2-mercapto-ethanol treatment was greater in some patients with a renal origin for their bacteriuria, and 22 of 39 with upper tract involvement and 12 of 40 with bladder bacteriuria (p<.025) had residual titers of 1:32 or greater.

Results of Maximal Urinary Concentration Studies

The results of maximum solution concentration (U_{max}) determined in 66 patients are summarized in Figure 3. With the technique employed in the present study, most normal individuals achieve a U_{max} greater than 900 mOsm/kg, and values of U_{max} below 800 mOsm/kg are considered abnormal and signify an impairment in the capacity to excrete a maximally concentrated urine. It can be seen that 24 of 31 patients with infection limited to the bladder had a U_{max} greater than 800 mOsm/kg. Eight of the 31 had a U_{max} greater than 1,000 mOsm/kg, and 16 more concentrated between 800 and 1,000 mOsm/kg. On

found in patients with infection confined to the bladder. However, titers equal to or greater than 1:512 were significantly more frequent (p<.05) in patients with renal bacteriuria; and titers in serum of 1:512 or greater were found against 10 of 39 organisms in patients with renal bacteriuria, whereas only one of 40 with infection in the lower tract had an antibody response of this magnitude. However, a titer in serum of 1:512 was an arbitrary distinction, and was the only value at which a significant difference was seen between patients with renal and bladder bacteriuria.

The results of residual hemagglutinating antibody titers found after addition of 2-mercaptoethanol are summarized in Figure 2. It can be seen that this procedure was no more discriminatory than tests of hemagglutinating activity in untreated serum. However, similar to the results observed with whole serum,

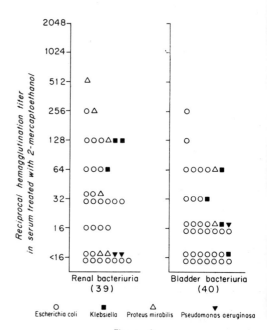

Figure 2

Reciprocal Hemagglutination Titers in Serum Treated with 2-Mercaptoethanol in Patients with Bacteriuria. (Reproduced with permission. Ref. 3.)

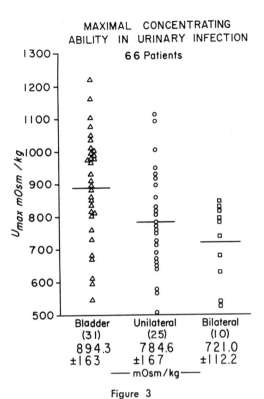

MAXIMAL CONCENTRATING
ABILITY IN URINARY INFECTION
66 Patients

Bladder (31)	Unilateral (25)	Bilateral (10)
894.3 ±163	784.6 ±167	721.0 ±112.2

— mOsm/kg —

Figure 3

Maximal Concentrating Ability in Patients with Recurrent Bacteriuria Correlated with the Site of Infection. (Reproduced with permission. Ref. 8.)

the other hand, 14 of 25 patients with unilateral infection and 7 of 10 with bilateral involvement failed to concentrate above 800 mOsm/kg. Furthermore, none of 10 patients with bilateral renal bacteriuria concentrated to 900 mOsm/kg. Comparing the mean values of U_{max} in bladder with renal bacteriuria, individuals with bladder infection (894 mOsm/kg) concentrated significantly better than patients with either unilateral (784 mOsm/kg) or bilateral (721 mOsm/kg) renal bacteriuria ($p<.025$, $p<.005$).

The results of differential U_{max} in 24 patients with bladder bacteriuria and 19 with unilateral infections studied during the period of maximal antidiuresis are summarized in Figure 4. Overall, there were no consistent differences between left and right kidneys among patients with bladder bacteriuria. On

the other hand, in patients with unilateral renal bacteriuria the infected kidney generally excreted urine with a lower U_{max} than did the noninfected side ($p<.005$). The difference exceeded 100 mOsm/kg in 13 of 19 patients with unilateral renal infection. Furthermore, only one patient with unilateral renal bacteriuria failed to achieve a more concentrated urine on the noninfected side.

Results of Urinary Beta-Glucuronidase Activity

The results of beta-glucuronidase activity determined in 21 patients with bladder bacteriuria, 25 patients with unilateral or bilateral renal bacteriuria, and 46 normal individuals, are summarized in Figure 5. The mean beta-glucuronidase activity in the urine of 46 control subjects was 5.1 ± 2.9 units with the accepted upper limit of normal (99% confidence limit) at 13.5 units. This did not differ significantly from the activities in urine of patients with bladder bacteriuria (6.6 ± 3.1 units) or renal bacteriuria (8.7 ± 5.3 units). Although not depicted in the Figure, 14 patients with unilateral renal bacteriuria had levels of activity in their urine comparable to 11 patients with bilateral involvement. Furthermore, the activity in urine from the infected side in patients with unilateral infection did not differ significantly from the activity in the noninfected side. Although four patients with renal bacteriuria (three with unilateral and one with bilateral infection) did demonstrate activity in their urine above 13.5 units, two of these patients had diabetic glomerulosclerosis, one had a renal calculus, and one was found to have a bladder carcinoma in addition to upper tract bacteriuria.

Discussion

The findings in these ongoing studies provide several pieces of information concerning the differentiation of renal from bladder bacteriuria in asymptomatic patients. Firstly, in general, patients with renal bacteriuria, either unilateral or bilateral, were found to have higher antibody titers than did patients with infection localized to the bladder. However, because of the wide range of titers, determination of hemagglutinating antibody activity was only of limited usefulness in predicting

147

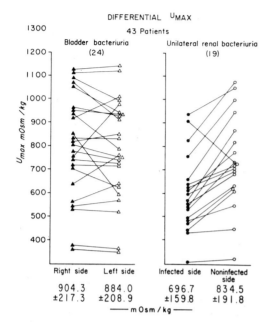

Figure 4

Differential Maximal Concentrating Ability in Patients with Bladder Bacteriuria and Patients with Unilateral Renal Infection. (Reproduced with permission. Ref. 8.)

the site of infection in individual patients with asymptomatic urinary tract infection. Perhaps, the main clinical application of determination of the serum antibody activity may be in epidemiologic and therapeutic studies of groups of patients with asymptomatic bacteriuria. Coupled with studies of maximal urinary concentrating ability, it remains possible that more sensitive and precise methods of determining antibody activity may be employed to select those patients more likely to have renal involvement.[6,7]

Secondly, our findings demonstrate that renal infection, even in the asymptomatic patient with normal or only slightly impaired creatinine clearances, often is associated with impairment of ability to excrete a maximally concentrated urine. These data also support the expectation that infection of the bladder per se generally is not associated with impaired concentrating ability. In addition,

other studies not reported herein have demonstrated an improvement in U_{max} following successful antibiotic treatment of renal but not bladder bacteriuria.[8] Furthermore, the observation that in unilateral upper-tract infection, the maximal concentration of urine was not reduced on the noninfected side, strongly implicates the presence of bacteria in the concentrating abnormality. It is conceivable that the mere presence of gram-negative microorganisms in the renal medulla may interfere with U_{max}, apart from causing any permanent destruction in renal mass or inciting any marked inflammatory response. Whatever ultimately is determined to be the cause of the concentrating defect, the results of our studies suggest that it is largely reversible with effective antimicrobial therapy and provide a rationale for treatment of patients with renal bacteriuria even when they are free of symptoms.

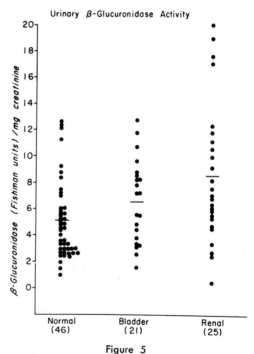

Figure 5

Urinary Beta-Glucuronidase Activity in Normal Subjects and Patients with Urinary Tract Infection. (Reproduced with permission. Ref. 5.)

Finally, the results of the present studies demonstrate that unlike the findings observed in patients with active pyelonephritis,[9] asymptomatic patients with renal bacteriuria do not have elevations of urinary beta-glucuronidase activity. An associated abnormality of the urinary tract or concomitant renal parenchymal disease was present in the only four patients in our study who did have elevated enzyme activity. In experimental models of pyelonephritis, elevations in the excretion of beta-glucuronidase were observed primarily in animals with severe inflammatory disease.[10] If these observations in experimental animals are applicable to the situation in man, it appears that most patients with asymptomatic bacteriuria emanating from the upper tract have a minimal inflammatory response in the renal parenchyma. However, it is also possible that asymptomatic patients defined as having upper tract infection by ureteral urine culture may have involvement only of the ureter or renal pelvis. If the infections were luminal or superficial, such patients might more closely resemble patients with infection confined to the bladder. In either case, it appears unlikely on the basis of these findings that determination of beta-glucuronidase activity will find much place in differentiating renal from bladder bacteriuria in most patients with urinary tract infection.

ACKNOWLEDGMENTS

Many physicians participated in the design, implementation, and interpretation of these studies. I would like particularly to express my appreciation to Dr. Allan R. Ronald and Dr. H. Clark for their splendid efforts in these studies.

REFERENCES

1. Stamey TA. Govan DE and Palmer JM: The localization and treatment of urinary tract infections: The role of bactericidal urine levels as opposed to serum levels. Medicine 44:1-36, 1965.
2. Turck M, Ronald AR and Petersdorf RG: Relapse and reinfection in chronic bacteriuria. II. The correlation between site of infection and pattern of recurrence in chronic bacteriuria. NEJM 278: 422-427, 1968.
3. Clark H. Ronald AR and Turck M: Serum antibody response in renal versus bladder bacteriuria. J Inf Dis, May 1971.
4. Ronald AR, Cutler RE and Turck M: Effect of bacteriuria on the renal concentrating mechanisms. Ann Int Med 70:723-733, 1969.
5. Ronald AR, Silverblatt F, Clark H, et al: Failure of urinary beta-glucuronidase activity to localize site of urinary tract infection. Appl Microbiol, 1971.
6. Norden CW, Levy PS and Kass EH: Predictive effect of urinary concentrating ability and hemagglutinating antibody titer upon response to antimicrobial therapy in bacteriuria of pregnancy. J Inf Dis 121:588-596, 1970.
7. Reeves DS and Brumfitt W: Localization of urinary tract infection. Urinary Tract Infection. O'Grady F and Brumfitt W ed, London, Oxford Univ Press 1968, p 53-67.
8. Clark H. Ronald AR, Cutler RE, et al: The correlation between site of infection and maximal concentrating ability in bacteriuria. J Inf Dis 120:47-51, 1969.
9. Bank N and Bailine SH: Urinary beta-glucuronidase activity in patients with urinary tract infection. NEJM 272:70-75, 1965.
10. Coonrod D and Paterson PY: Urinary beta-glucuronidase in renal injury. II. Excretion patterns in experimental staphylococcal pyelonephritis in rats. J Lab Clin Med 73:17-24, 1969.

THE DIAGNOSIS AND MANAGEMENT OF
URINARY INFECTION IN FEMALES

● Urinary tract infections occur frequently in female patients and present a wide spectrum of clinical syndromes. Recognition of such infection and localization in the urinary tract are important for successful treatment.

ALLAN R. RONALD, M.D.

Bacterial infections of the urinary tract in adult females are among the commonest indications for antimicrobial therapy in medical practice. Whereas most acute infections are self-limited, urinary infections frequently persist and recur, despite multiple urologic procedures and extensive prolonged therapeutic regimens. This review is concerned with an approach to the investigation and treatment of urinary infection in females that, if followed, may result in more rational management.

Prevalence Studies

Prevalence studies in healthy populations have delineated segments of the population with an increased risk of urinary infection. In school age and adolescent girls, several studies have consistently given prevalence rates between 1 and 2%.[1] With marriage, the prevalence rate increases to between 3 and 6%.[2] Although parity has a minimal effect on increasing prevalence, many infections become symptomatic with pregnancy.[3] The prevalence is higher in women from lower socioeconomic groups.[4] Surprisingly, nuns have a frequency of bacteriuria much lower than their married counterparts.[2]

During 1970, 621 women were surveyed for bacteriuria at the time of their first prenatal visit to the Winnipeg General Hospital Prenatal Clinic. The prevalence of urinary infec-

Dr. Ronald is Assistant Professor, Departments of Medical Microbiology and Medicine, University of Manitoba and the Winnipeg General Hospital, Winnipeg, Manitoba, Canada.

tion, in most instances proven by catheterization, was unusually high with a rate of 9.8%. This population was further categorized into 176 of Indian ethnic origin and 445 who were not of Indian origin. The former group had a very high prevalence of 17.6%. This contrasts with a prevalence of 7.6% in the non-Indian population. No obvious explanation is known to account for the higher prevalence of bacteriuria in Indian population in this survey. Further studies are under way to document this prevalence and determine its significance.

Diagnosis

The diagnosis of urinary infection depends upon the demonstration of significant numbers of bacteria in a urine collected without extraurinary contamination. Fortunately for purposes of diagnosis, most patients with infection have greater than 100,000 organisms/ml. Female patients, especially those with gram-negative colonization of their perineum, often have voided urine with low counts, usually less than 10,000. In order to obtain maximum value from this differential, continued emphasis must be placed on proper collection and transport of urine cultures.

In alert, cooperative patients, a clean voided midstream urine is quite satisfactory if the patient understands the technique and is supervised. A single clean voided urine culture with $>10^5$ organisms/ml is about 80% accurate in predicting urinary infection. Two consecutive clean voided urine cultures containing the same pathogen in significant amounts increase the accuracy of diagnosis to almost 95%. In patients with unequivocal symptoms of acute urinary infection, one urine is adequate. However, in surveys and in the care of patients with low grade or asymptomatic infection, a second confirmatory culture should be obtained before initiating therapy. Gram-positive organisms other than enterococci are rarely true urinary pathogens and should be confirmed by serial cultures or a catheterized sample. At room temperature, organisms in urine can double every 30 minutes. A few contaminants can quickly increase to 'significant' numbers. Unless the culture is planted immediately, refrigeration following collection is mandatory. Fortunately, most urinary pathogens are relatively hardy and survive at 4°C for 8 to 12 hours without any change in colony count or viability.

Localization of Infection

The localization of infection to exclude renal involvement in patients with no symptoms or lower tract symptoms only is increasingly important. Patients with renal infection are at greater risk from their disease and require more extensive investigation and prolonged therapy. The neomycin bladder washout test first described by Fairley[5,6] readily permits the localization of infection in female patients. This procedure is simple, does not require special urologic skills, and can be carried out by a nurse or other paramedical personnel. The bacteriologic techniques are those routinely used in most laboratories. In over 90% of the patients, interpretation of the results is straightforward. This test should be available to all physicians treating patients with recurrent urinary infection.

The urinary bladder is temporarily 'sterilized' following the neomycin bladder washout test. To our surprise, many patients were cured of their infection following localization without additional antimicrobial therapy. To date, of 49 patients with bladder infection only, 20 have been cured of that infection by the localization procedure.

The ease of eradicating bladder infection

in females has suggested to us a therapeutic method to differentiate renal from bladder infection. Following localization with the neomycin bladder washout test, the patient was followed for recurrence of urinary infection. Patients cured with this test were not treated unless infection recurred. However, patients whose infection persisted were given a single injection of 500 mg of kanamycin. Eighty-seven patients have been studied to date. Thirty-five had lower infection by the localization technique. Thirty of these patients were cured with kanamycin. Five immediately relapsed with the same bacterial pathogen. The remaining fifty-two patients had renal infection. Thirty-six patients relapsed all within a few days of receiving kanamycin. Surprisingly, 16 patients with infection emanating from their ureters were cured with a single injection of kanamycin. Overall, of 41 patients who relapsed after kanamycin, 36 had upper tract infection. That is, seven of eight patients were correctly predicted by this diagnostic test to have renal infection. This means of differentiating renal from bladder infection deserves further study and may be a simple method for routine use in office practice.

Therapy of Urinary Infection

Urinary infections were adequately treated in most instances prior to the discovery of antimicrobics. Fluid, analgesics and bed rest usually resulted in rapid symptomatic relief. At present, 'wonder drugs' are often given unwarranted credit by both patients and physicians.

Several general principles are useful guidelines in the selection of an antimicrobic and the duration of therapy.

First, symptomatic relief correlates poorly with bacteriologic results. Infection often persists despite clinical improvement. For ultimate success, eradication of bacteria is more important than immediate symptomatic improvement. A urine culture should be obtained during therapy to assess the *in vivo* sensitivity to the antimicrobic and ensure that the organism has been eradicated.

Second, over 90% of uncomplicated acute urinary infections are caused by *Escherichia*

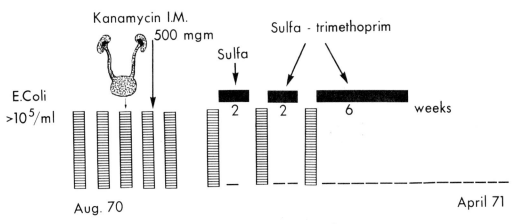

Figure 1 Recurrent relapsing urinary infection.

coli. A great many agents can successfully treat these infections, and the choice depends upon cost, side effects, mode of administration, individual idiosyncrasies, and the physician's personal experience. Few controlled studies are available conclusively showing one agent to be better than others if the infecting organism is eradicated during therapy.

Third, indiscriminate prolongation of therapy should not be routinely used in patients with repeated infection. If infection recurs following effective therapy, the site of origin of bacteriuria determines the duration of subsequent therapy. Prolonged therapy will not prevent multiple bladder reinfections and may alter the patient's bacterial ecology so that subsequent reinfections will be resistant to the drug the patient has been taking.

Specific therapeutic regimens for urinary infection will be discussed under the following headings:

1. acute pyelonephritis
2. acute cystitis & asymptomatic bacteriuria
3. recurrent bacteriuria
4. complicated urinary infection

Acute pyelonephritis: The patient is usually ill with flank pain, chills, and fever and may have bacteremia accompanying renal invasion. Hospital admission for initial therapy is usually indicated. An abdominal film is useful to exclude renal calculi and to check renal size. Renal function should be assessed with a BUN. Papillary necrosis frequently accompanies acute pyelonephritis, particularly in patients with a history of diabetes or analgesic abuse. Patients with acute pyelonephritis occasionally develop large cortical abscesses or a perinephric abscess that may require surgical drainage.

Optimal antimicrobial therapy for acute pyelonephritis should initially be administered parenterally. Ampicillin (1 gm q6h I.V.) or kanamycin (500 mg q12h I.M.) are the drugs of choice although sulphonamides still have some use. The patient should be afebrile by 72 hours and oral therapy with either ampicillin or nitrofurantoin continued for two weeks. A culture is obtained one week after therapy is completed and again in one month. In the absence of upper tract pathology, relapse (recurrence with the same bacterial pathogen) occurs in less than 10% of patients. Pyelography should be done during convalescence.

Acute cystitis and asymptomatic bacteriuria:

153

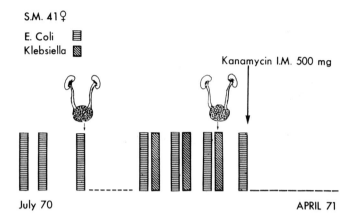

S.M. 41♀

E. Coli

Klebsiella

Kanamycin I.M. 500 mg

Figure 2

Recurrent reinfecting urinary infection.

July 70

APRIL 71

Although temporarily distressing acute cystitis is usually a benign, self-limiting disease. However, if upper tract infection is present, further investigations and therapy are warranted. As discussed previously, we feel the simplest method to diagnose renal infection, is follow-up after a short course of therapy (three to five days) with an effective antimicrobic. A culture should be obtained during therapy to ensure eradication of infection. Oral agents are adequate, and one of the sulphonamides or nitrofurantoin is the therapy of choice. Whenever short-term therapy is used, follow-up cultures must be obtained in order to diagnose the patient with renal infection.

Recurrent infection: Despite eradication of infection during therapy, 20 to 60% of female patients will have recurrences sometime within a year following treatment. Many infections are asymptomatic and will be detected only if routine follow-up cultures are obtained. Rapid recurrences with the same organism (relapse) require a thorough assessment to rule out curable surgical lesions. Pyelography, cysto-urethrography, and sometimes cystoscopy may disclose congenital abnormalities. These studies should be done well initially with the first recurrence and should not be repeated unnecessarily.

Figure 1 depicts a patient with recurrent asymptomatic *E. coli* bacteriuria with the same strain, who had upper tract infection

by localization and relapsed after kanamycin. She relapsed on two further occasions after short courses of antimicrobial therapy. The infection was finally eradicated with six weeks of therapy. Although no controlled evidence is available, six weeks of nalidixic acid has in our experience been particularly effective in patients with parenchymal renal infection.

Figure 2 presents a patient with a reinfecting recurrence. This 41-year-old pregnant female had a persistent bladder *E. coli* infection for several months. It was eradicated by the neomycin bladder washout test. Subsequently two months later, she recurred with urine cultures positive for both *E. coli* and *Klebsiella*. In our experience, double infections are unusual and should be documented with repeated cultures. On this occasion, localization again showed that both organisms were confined to the bladder. The *Klebsiella* was eradicated with the neomycin bladder washout, but the *E. coli* persisted and was not eradicated until the patient was given 500 mg of I.M. kanamycin. She has had no recurrences since. This patient demonstrates the ease of eradication of bladder infection in females. Most recurrences due to reinfections will respond to repeated short courses of chemotherapy. If these recurrences are infrequent, no specific measures other than an annual urine culture are necessary. For patients with several recurrences each year, preventive measures should be attempted. Currently, we recommend urinary acidification with ascorbic acid and methenamine mandelate to maintain an early morning urinary pH of 5.5. This presumably discourages bacterial growth in the urine and prevents reinfections. Patients whose reinfections appear to follow sexual exposure may be helped by one dose of prophylactic antimicrobic taken prior to intercourse. A tablet of penicillin 250 mg or nitrofurantoin 50 mg is an inexpensive regimen. Patients should also be instructed to void following intercourse.

Complicated urinary-infection: Patients with congenital urinary anomalies or neurogenic bladders with large residual urines cannot be treated satisfactorily with any drug regimens. Continuous 'suppressive' sulphonamide regimens are useful for patients with surgically irreparable lesions and may retard renal deterioration. Acute symptomatic flare-ups occur in these patients and should be treated with short courses of antimicrobic to which the organism is susceptible. If possible, a more susceptible organism should not be eradicated from the urinary tracts in these patients as 'success' will only result in replacement with more resistant organisms, particularly *Pseudomonas*.

Conclusions

Study of urinary infection in females can be rewarding combining bacteriologic principles with clinical skills. Although they frequently recur, the principles of management outlined in this review can provide a rational approach to a difficult problem.

ACKNOWLEDGEMENTS

I would like to thank Mrs. Kathe Stagno, the study coordinator, Joan Wilkie who performed the localizations and Claudette Cates who did the bacteriology. Also, my thanks to the outpatient staff at the Women's Pavilion, Winnipeg General Hospital. This investigation was supported by the Medical Research Council (Canada) grant MA 3065.

REFERENCES

1. Kunin CM: Epidemiology and natural history of urinary tract infection in school age children. Ped Clin N Am 18:509, 1971.
2. Kunin CM and McCormack RC: Bacteriuria and blood pressure among nuns and working women. NEJM 278:635, 1968.
3. Savage WE, Hajj SM and Kass EH: Demographic and prognostic characteristics of bacteriuria in pregnancy. Med 46: 385, 1967.
4. Turck M, Goffe BS and Petersdorf RG: Bacteriuria of pregnancy, relation to socioeconomic factors. NEJM 266:857, 1962.
5. Fairley KF, Bond AG, Brown RB, et al: Simple test to determine the site eo urinary tract infection. Lancet 2:427, 1967.
6. Boutros P, Mourtada H and Ronald AR: Urinary infection localization. Antimicrobial Agents & Chemo, 1970. In press.

METABOLISM AND LABORATORY STUDIES WITH INDANYL CARBENICILLIN

● A new ester of carbenicillin appears to be resistant to gastric acid. After oral administration therapeutic levels of the antibiotic are present in the urine.

KENNETH BUTLER, Ph.D.
ARTHUR R. ENGLISH, Ph.D.
A. K. KNIRSCH, M.D.
J. J. KORST, Ph.D.

Carbenicillin indanyl sodium is N-(2-carboxy-3, 3-dimethyl-7-oxo-4-thia-1-azabicyclo [3.2.0] hept-6-yl)-2-phenylmalonamic acid 5-indanyl ester, sodium salt, a new semi-synthetic penicillin. It is an acid-stable and readily absorbed derivative of carbenicillin, ie, one in which the original biologically active component is rendered useful for oral administration by masking a polar functional group of the parent drug to produce a more lipid soluble compound. In the case of carbenicillin indanyl sodium, this polar functional group is the α-carboxylic acid moiety of carbenicillin which is bound through ester linkage to 5-indanol.

Materials and Methods

In vitro studies. Carbenicillin indanyl sodium was used in the form of the crystalline mono-sodium salt, carbenicillin was used in the form of the amorphous disodium salt, and ampicillin was used as the trihydrate. The various micro-organisms utilized were either stock cultures that had been maintained in this laboratory for a number of years or fresh clinical isolates from hospitals in different geographical locations.

Tests of *in vitro* susceptibility were done by the conventional 2-fold serial dilution technique in Brain-Heart Infusion broth (Pfizer Diagnostics). The inoculum consisted of 0.5 ml of a 1 X10^{-3} dilution of an overnight culture

incubated at 37 C. The tests were carried out in plastic DisPoso Trays (Linbro Chemical Co., New Haven), total final volume in each cup being 1 ml. The test was read visually, the minimal inhibitory concentration (MIC) being the lowest concentration of antibiotic preventing visual turbidity after overnight incubation of the culture at 37 C.

In vitro acid stability studies. A penicillin at 400 or 800 mcg/ml was added to synthetic gastric juice (pH 2.0), and the solution was maintained for one hour in a 37 C water bath. A 0.5 ml portion was serially diluted in B.H.I. broth through ten tubes and the tubes inoculated with 0.5 ml of a suitably diluted culture of *Staphylococcus aureus*. MIC values were read after incubation at 37 C for approximately 20 hours and compared with regular MIC values against the same test organism. The percentage loss of biological activity was calculated from the differences of MIC values.

In vivo studies. Experimental systemic infections were produced in mice by intraperitoneal inoculation of standardized bacterial cultures suspended in 5% hog gastric mucin.

Dr. Butler is Manager, Antibiotics for Human Infectious Diseases, Charles Pfizer and Company.

157

	Minimum Inhibitory Concentration mcg/ml (median values)		
	CP-15,464-2	Carbeni- cillin	Ampi- cillin
Staphylococcus aureus (5)	0.19	0.78	0.02
Staphylococcus aureus (400;)	25	12.5	200
Streptococcus pyogenes (8668)	0.0025	0.19	0.005
Streptococcus pyogenes (C203)	0.0012	0.19	0.002
Streptococcus faecalis	0.045	3.12	0.01
Diplococcus pneumoniae	0.02	0.39	0.002
Aerobacter aerogenes	3.12	6.25	100
Escherichia coli	3.12	3.12	3.12
Proteus vulgaris	3.12	3.12	3.12
Proteus mirabilis	1.56	1.56	3.12
Proteus rettgeri	12.5	3.12	200
Proteus morgani	12.5	6.25	>200
Pseudomonas (10490)	1.56	0.78	25
Pseudomonas aeruginosa (173)	50	75	>200
Salmonella typhosa	12.5	12.5	3.12
Klebsiella pneumoniae (132)	3.12	12.5	1.56
Klebsiella pneumoniae	200	3.12	—
Vibrio comma	3.12	200	1.56
Pasteurella multocida	0.19	0.09	0.09
Shigella sonnei	6.25	12.5	6.25

Table 1

IN VITRO ANTIBACTERIAL
ACTIVITY AGAINST SELECTED
BACTERIAL SPECIES

The severity of infection was consistently at 1-10 LD 100, ie, 1-10 times the number of organisms needed to kill 100% of the mice under the conditions of the experiment. The dose of antibiotic required to protect 50% of the mice (PD$_{50}$) was calculated in each experiment at 96 hours after challenge by use of a probit method.[1]

Experimental disease of the urinary tract in rats was produced with *Pseudomonas aeruginosa* 173, *Proteus vulgaris* 59 and *Escherichia coli* 028. The basic details of the technique used to produce infections with *P. vul-*garis and *P. aeruginosa* have been published previously in detail.[2] When the *E. coli* model was used, the infection was produced by ureter-ligation followed by intravenous administration of the infecting organism. In all instances, infected rats were treated orally once a day for eight days; the first dose was administered one day after challenge. Rats were sacrificed after completion of therapy, kidneys were removed and macerated, and the number of viable organisms was determined by plate counting. Such counts are expressed as the log average of the viable count.

Table 2

CARBENICILLIN INDANYL SODIUM; ACTIVITY AGAINST CLINICAL ISOLATES

	Number of Isolates	Antibiotic	Cumulative Percent Susceptibility:							>200 mcg/ml
			3.12 and <	6.25	12.5	25	50	100	200	
Pseudomonas aeruginosa	48	Indanyl Carbenicillin	4%	4%	8%	21%	29%	56%	69%	100%
		Carbenicillin	10%	19%	21%	25%	44%	73%	90%	100%
Proteus Indolepositive	48	Indanyl Carbenicillin	0%	45%	73%	100%				
		Carbenicillin	54%	54%	73%	73%	73%	100%		
Proteus mirabilis	9	Indanyl Carbenicillin	0%	44%	89%	100%				
		Carbenicillin	56%	89%	100%					
Escherichia coli	50	Indanyl Carbenicillin	16%	60%	92%	96%	96%	96%	98%	100%
		Carbenicillin	6%	18%	72%	80%	94%	96%	96%	100%

Antibiotic Assay Procedures.

The concentration of carbenicillin in serum samples was determined by a 5 cup cylinder plate assay with a double layer of agar (a layer of agar inoculated with *Pseudomonas aeruginosa NCTC* 10490 on top of a layer of plain agar). The sensitivity of this assay is 3-4 mcg/ml of carbenicillin in serum; this is the *standard* carbenicillin bio-assay. The standard curve for carbenicillin indanyl sodium closely resembles that for carbenicillin in this assay procedure, probably because of hydrolysis of the derivative to produce carbenicillin under the assay conditions. However, the levels of carbenicillin indanyl sodium in serum actually observed after oral dosage were too low to be detected by this method.

Differential Assay Procedure for carbenicillin and carbenicillin indanyl sodium in serum.

To 1.0 ml of serum was added 2 ml of reagent grade acetone to produce a heavy precipitate of serum proteins. The mixture was stirred intermittently with a rod for ten minutes, then filtered through a sintered glass funnel. The cake was washed well with small volumes of acetone and the filtrate and washings were combined (total volume circa 15 ml). To the acetone solution was added 1.0

	MIC (mcg/ml), Median Values; *Staphylococcus Aureus*		
	BHI(pH 7.2)	Gastric Juice pH 2.0	% Loss of Activity at pH 2.0
Carbenicillin Indanyl Sodium	0.09	0.09	0%
Carbenicillin- Disodium	1.56	200	99.2%
Benzyl penicillin	0.06	200	99.9%

TABLE 3

STABILITY OF CARBENICILLIN INDANYL SODIUM IN SYNTHETIC GASTRIC JUICE AT 37 C FOR ONE HOUR

TABLE 4

In vivo ACTIVITY OF CARBENICILLIN INDANYL SODIUM IN ACUTE SYSTEMIC INFECTIONS
IN MICE

PD_{50} mg/kg (calculated on a penicillin, free-acid basis)
with 95% Confidence Limits

| | CP-15,464-2 | | Carbenicillin | Ampicillin |
	Oral	S. C.	S. C.	Oral
Escherichia coli	20.5 ± 6.1	22 ± 5.9	21.5 ± 5.9	25 ± 13
Staphylococcus aureus	40 ± 10.7	41 ± 9.8	38 ± 3.1	—
Streptococcus pyogenes	14 ± 4.5	8 ± 2.5	8.7 ± 2.7	—
Proteus species				
P. vulgaris	190		200 ± 61	>400
P. mirabilis	175		185 ± 88	200 ± 80
Pseudomonas aeruginosa				
Strain — JH47	250 ± 135		200 ± 98	>400
A38	290		210 ± 84	>400

gm of silicic acid, and the mixture was swirled intermittently for twenty minutes. After this time the mixture was again filtered and the silicic acid was washed well with small volumes of acetone (total volume circa 35 ml). The combined filtrate and washings were evaporated under reduced pressure to a partially solid residue. The residue was dissolved in 0.25 ml of methanol, and the solution was spotted at three levels (5, 10, 20 lambda) on a thin layer chromatographic (TLC) plate (Eastman Chromagram-Sheet 6060 — Silica Gel with fluorescent indicator) along with three levels of a control. The plate was developed (300 parts acetone: 50 parts of a 0.2*M* aqueous sodium acetate solution), then plated on a *B. subtilis* bioplate for fifteen minutes. The TLC sheets were removed from the agar, and the bioplates were developed overnight at 37 C. From the comparison of the sizes of the zones of inhibition from the sample with those of the known control, an estimate was made of the drug concentration in the sample.

1. The volume of serum used is dependent upon the concentration of drug in the serum. In the range of 10-20 mcg/ml, 1 ml of serum is adequate. In the 5 mcg/ml range or less, 2.0 ml of serum should be used. If 2.0 ml of serum is used, 4 ml of acetone should be added. Also the cake should be washed with a correspondingly greater amount of acetone and 2.0 gm of silicic acid should be added to the filtrate.

2. The transfer during the filtration and subsequent wash of the cake must be quantitative.

3. The silicic acid removes an additional amount of protein.

4. The levels spotted on the TLC plates must be such that a difference in concentration will be readily discernible. If there is too much drug in the spots, all will be very intense, ie, give large zones of inhibition and no reasonable estimate of relative concentration can be made. Hence, the lower level must afford a very weak zone, or no zone.

5. The control is a sample of serum spiked with the drug in question at a level approximating the anticipated serum level.

		Dosage	Log viable organisms/ gram kidney	
		mg/kg	Treated	Inf. Control
Escherichia coli	Carbenicillin Indanyl Sodium	50	1.32	7.63
		25	2.27	7.63
		12.5	3.47	7.63
	Carbenicillin (subcut.)	50	1.52	6.76
	Cephalexin (oral)	50	2.88	8.15
	Cephalo-glycin (oral)	200	6.64	7.35
	Ampicillin (oral)	50	1.37	6.76
Pseudomonas aeruginosa	Carbenicillin Indanyl Sodium	100	2.89	5.72
	Carbenicillin (subcut.)	100	3.57	5.72
	Ampicillin (oral)	100	5.30	5.72
Proteus vulgaris	Carbenicillin Indanyl Sodium	50	3.08	6.57
	Carbenicillin (subcut.)	50	4.42	5.72
	Furadantin (oral)	50	2.35	6.57

TABLE 5

ACTIVITY OF CARBENICILLIN INDANYL SODIUM AGAINST URINARY TRACT INFECTIONS IN RATS

This control is worked up in exactly the same manner as the test sample.

6. The bioplate is prepared from Streptomycin assay agar (with yeast extract) prepared according to the standard directions. For one plate (38x48 cm), 300 ml of agar broth seeded with *B. subtilis* was used. Plates were poured on a level surface to insure uniform thickness of the agar layer. This is necessary since the size of the zone of inhibition is a function of the agar thickness.

Results and Discussion

Carbenicillin is a recently introduced semi-synthetic penicillin which has found wide application for the treatment of gram-negative infections. It is, however, a very polar substance and not stable in acidic solutions; at pH 2.0 it has a half-life of less than thirty minutes, and it is readily destroyed by gastric juice. Therefore, this antibiotic is not effective when administered by the oral route. Carbenicillin indanyl sodium was prepared in an attempt to overcome these deficiencies and yet retain the desirable biological properties of carbenicillin. This particular carbenicillin ester was selected from a large number of homologs that had been synthesized based upon considerations of overall performance *in*

TABLE 6
SINGLE DOSE STUDY WITH CARBENICILLIN INDANYL SODIUM IN HUMAN VOLUNTEERS*

Drug	Dose	Serum carbenicillin levels (mcg/ml) free acid						Urinary Excretion — % of administered dose			
		Hours after Dose						Hours after Dose			
		0	½	1	2	3	4	0-3	3-6	6-24	24-
Carbenicillin	250 mg	0	3.3	3.1	2.6	0	0	23.2	16.4	6.5	0
(i.m.)	500 mg	0	15.0	14.5	9.3	4.3	0	20.9	12.0	18.5	0
Carbenicillin	500 mg	0	2.1	4.9	0	0	0	18.3	12.0	3.0	0
Indanyl	1000 mg	0	8.3	10.2	7.5	3.1	0	13.4	15.8	10.3	0
Sodium											

*These data are the average values obtained for twelve subjects.

vitro and *in vivo* and favorable toxicological properties. The use of an indanyl ester provides chemical stability which prevents acid-catalyzed degradation by gastric juice; it also provides the lipophilic properties necessary for good absorption from the gastrointestinal tract. The temporary role of the phenolic indanol moiety is to aid the oral absorption of the parent drug; it is removed *in vivo* regenerating the active principal (carbenicillin) and metabolic by-products derived from 5-indanol.

In vitro studies. Both carbenicillin indanyl sodium and carbenicillin have relatively broad spectra of activity against gram-positive and gram-negative bacteria. A sample study carried out in these laboratories is shown in Table 1. Further *in vitro* data for carbenicillin and its indanyl ester against a series of gram-negative clinical isolates are displayed in Table 2. In general, the *in vitro* profile of carbenicillin indanyl sodium closely resembles that of carbenicillin and shows good activity against indole positive *Proteus* and *Pseudomonas* species. The enhanced *in vitro* potency of the indanyl ester against certain gram-positive bacteria as compared to carbenicillin is the result of the less acidic properties and the increased lipophilic character of the ester. These physical-chemical properties of penicillins have a profound effect upon the uptake and binding of the antibiotics to the gram-positive bacterial cells. Similar effects were not observed in gram-negative bacteria, probably because of hydrolysis of the ester during the incubation period. It should be noted that the improved gram-positive activity of carbenicillin indanyl sodium is not manifested in *in vivo* situations; the drug is so rapidly metabolized following oral absorption that it produces the same biological response as carbenicillin.

The chemical stability of carbenicillin indanyl sodium is illustrated in Table 3. The percent degradation was obtained from MIC values determined after the antibiotics had been incubated with synthetic gastric juice (pH 2.0) for one hour at 37 C. The indanyl ester of carbenicillin was quite stable, but both carbenicillin and benzyl penicillin were almost totally destroyed under these experimental conditions.

In vivo studies. The indanyl ester of carbenicillin proved to be as effective when administered orally as when given by the subcutaneous route for the treatment of acute experimental infections in mice. (Table 4) The PD_{50} values are expressed in terms of mg/kg of the penicillin salt; those for indanyl carbenicillin (CP-15,464) have not been adjusted to correct for the increased molecular weight resulting from the indanyl moiety. Thus, on a weight for weight basis, the indanyl ester is as active *in vivo* as carbenicillin, even though it contains only 76% by weight

TABLE 7

MULTIPLE DOSE COMPARISON OF CARBENICILLIN INDANYL SODIUM AND AMPICILLIN IN HUMAN VOLUNTEERS

Antibiotic/ Dosage Regimen	Day of Test	Serum antibiotic levels (mcg/ml)* following first two doses of each day.									
		0	0.5	1	2	3	4	6	6.5	7	8
Ampicillin 500mg every 6 hours	1	0.0	0.81	2.22	2.16	0.95	0.45	0.15	0.40	1.55	1.27
	2	0.31	0.32	1.51	2.43	—	—	0.31	0.56	1.11	1.55
	3	0.29	0.34	0.50	0.81	0.40	0.26	0.07	0.05	0.85	1.23
	4	0.25	0.33	0.76	0.99		—	0.16	0.14	0.53	0.47
Carbenicillin Indanyl Sodium 500mg every 6 hours	1+	0.0	0.00 (<0.31)	2.53 (<0.31)	0.00 (<0.31)	0.0	0.0	0.0 —	3.18 (1.0)	6.31 (0.2)	4.75
	2	0.0	6.60 (1.0)	9.14 (0.2)	4.98 (<0.31)	—	—	0.0	6.78 (0.62)	6.61 (<0.31)	3.72
	3	0.0	6.16 (0.26)	11.0 (0.13)	6.07 (<0.31)	2.09	1.64	0.0	5.19 (0.28)	13.3 (0.1)	8.81
	4	0.0	3.02 (<0.31)	7.78 (<0.31)	8.34 (<0.31)	—	—	0.0	7.91 (0.31)	11.5 (<0.31)	8.79
Carbenicillin Indanyl Sodium 1000mg every 6 hours	1+	0.0	3.50 (0.2)	6.13 (0.2)	3.36 (0.62)	3.69	0.0	0.0	5.90 (0.73)	10.8 (0.52)	9.9
	2	0.0	5.71 (0.20)	11.9 (<0.62)	11.8 (0.83)	—	—	—	4.89 (<0.62)	9.81 (<0.62)	10.6
	3	1.04	9.44 (1.25)	18.0 (0.94)	11.3 (<0.62)	10.9	5.73	0.0	4.18 (<0.62)	13.8 (0.52)	15.1
	4	1.86	12.8 (1.1)	17.9 (0.57)	16.1 (0.41)	—	—	0.0	6.52 (0.20)	13.1 (<0.62)	16.0

*Values in parentheses and serum levels of carbenicillin indanyl sodium.
+The first dose of these studies was one-half of the presented regimen.

of carbenicillin as the biologically active component. The indanyl ester of carbenicillin had activity comparable with ampicillin when administered by the oral route for treatment of the systemic *E. coli* infections, and the orally administered ester was as effective as parenteral carbenicillin.

Both carbenicillin and its indanyl ester are effective agents for the treatment of experimental infections of the urinary tract in rats. Infections were produced by surgical methods, and the performance of an antibiotic was judged by its ability to reduce the count of viable organisms in the kidneys. In these experimental studies, oral carbenicillin indanyl sodium was compared with parenteral carbenicillin and with other orally effective agents which are commonly used for the treatment of urinary tract infections (ampicillin, cephalexin, cephaloglycin and Furadantin). Results are summarized in Table 5. Carbenicillin indanyl sodium was as effective as ampicillin and better than the other oral agents for the treatment of the *E. coli* infections as indicated by the reduction of the numbers of viable micro-organisms in the infected kidney tissues. Carbenicillin indanyl sodium was clearly superior to ampicillin in the *Pseudomonas* tests and comparable with Furadantin in the *Proteus vulgaris* infection. In all of these experimental urinary tract infections the effectiveness of the oral carbenicillin ester was generally as good as or better than that of parenteral carbenicillin.

TABLE 8

MULTIPLE DOSE COMPARISON OF CARBENICILLIN INDANYL SODIUM AND
AMPICILLIN: URINARY ANTIBIOTIC CONCENTRATION IN HUMAN VOLUNTEERS

Antibiotic	Dosage Regimen	Urine Antibiotic levels (mcg/ml) hrs. after commencing study											102-110
		0-3	3-6	6-24	24-27	27-30	30-48	48-51	51-54	54-72	72-75	75-78	78-96	
Ampicillin	500mg every 6 hours	219.2	164.6	125.8	182.5	171.4	114.0	470.8	58.1	256.5	321.7	225.0	178.7	90
Carbenicillin Indanyl Sodium	500 mg every 6 hours	455.0	67.0	518.4	697.5	117.1	437.8	756.6	355.5	543.3	444.5	387.9	284.4	46
	1000 mg every 6 hours	1162.6	272.3	655.3	602.1	71.3	780.1	818.9	607.6	151.0	599.8	183.6	441.0	47

Pharmacokinetics and Metabolism

Single and multiple dose studies with carbenicillin indanyl sodium were conducted with human volunteers. Serum and urine samples were carefully monitored to establish both the quantity and the identity of the biologically active components. For this purpose, a differential assay was developed to determine indanyl carbenicillin concentrations in the presence of both benzyl penicillin and carbenicillin. The method involved the separation of antibiotics in the mixture by thin layer chromatography and then assaying each biologically active component by a twofold serial dilution method on bioplates (test organism, *B. subtilis*). Results were obtained by an "end-point method" using appropriate control samples of known concentrations or by constructing standard curves from the diameters of the zones of inhibition. The end-point assay seemed to be the more dependable method

When assaying serum samples, it was first necessary to remove serum protein prior to the chromatographic separation of biologically active solutes. The procedure involved (i) precipitation of all serum proteins by use of an acetone/silicic acid treatment followed by (ii) evaporation of the filtrate to obtain the antibiotic activity in a concentrated form. [This assay method permitted recovery of

better than 85% of carbenicillin indanyl sodium from spiked serum samples. Recovery of carbenicillin was lower (20%), but since the quantity recovered was consistent from experiment to experiment, an accurate quantitation of carbenicillin content was achieved by use of appropriate controls. In practice, the standard cylinder-plate assay was used to determine the carbenicillin concentrations, and the differential assay was used to quantitate the indanyl ester and to corroborate the findings of the plate assay]. The concentrated antibiotic fraction was reconstituted in a small volume of solvent, and known aliquots of this solution were applied to a TLC plate. In theory, it requires only a MIC quantity of antibiotic to produce a zone of inhibition of the bioplates. This assay procedure is laborious but very sensitive and precise. It is possible to quantitate concentrations of indanyl carbenicillin in serum as low as 0.1 mcg/ml and even lower concentrations of benzyl penicillin.

Results of the single dose and multiple dose studies with carbenicillin indanyl sodium are shown in Tables 6, 7, and 8. Blood samples were processed immediately after collection, and serum samples were kept frozen until assayed (within three to four hours after processing). Under these conditions there was essentially no hydrolysis of carbenicillin in-

Antibiotic	Regimen	Antibiotic serum levels		Carbenicillin ester serum levels	
		Mean Peak Level (mcg/ ml)	Time after dose (hours)	Mean Peak level (mcg/ml)	Time after dose
Ampicillin	500mg, q.i.d.	1.41	1.6 hours	—	—
Carbenicillin Indanyl Sodium	500mg, q.i.d.*	9.37	1.14 hours	0.41	0.68 hours
	1000mg, q.i.d.*	14.92	1.14 hours	0.57	0.68 hours

*These values do not include the first dose of each study which were one half of the prescribed regimen.

TABLE 9

COMPARISON OF CARBENICILLIN INDANYL SODIUM AND AMPICILLIN PEAK SERUM LEVELS

danyl sodium to produce carbenicillin; thus the antibiotic titer shown in Tables 6 and 7 fairly represent what was present in serum at the time of collection. The single dose study was a comparison of tablets of carbenicillin indanyl sodium and parenteral carbenicillin. The serum antibiotic concentrations provided by parenteral carbenicillin are quite similar to those produced by twice the dosage of the carbenicillin indanyl ester. Again, it must be noted that the dosage regimen represents the weight of *indanyl carbenicillin-free acid* although the antibiotic was administered as the sodium salt and these numbers have not been adjusted to accommodate the differences in molecular weight between carbenicillin and its indanyl ester. Thus a 1000 mg dosage of the ester is equivalent to 764 mg of carbenicillin.

It is of interest to note that the blood levels of carbenicillin following oral dosage of the carbenicillin ester (14 mg/kg) in man compare favorably with those produced by 130 mg/kg in dogs.

The multiple dose study in human volunteers (Table 7) was a comparison of carbenicillin indanyl sodium at 500 mg and at 1000 mg four times a day with ampicillin (500 mg four times a day). The two groups receiving carbenicillin indanyl sodium consisted of six

men each; the group on ampicillin had five volunteers. The antibiotics were administered at regular six-hour intervals for four consecutive days, but the serum antibiotic levels were monitored only during the first eight hours of each day. The very first dose of the carbenicillin indanyl sodium regimens was one-half of the prescribed dosage. Good dose-response curves were obtained. Almost all of the active antibiotic in serum was carbenicillin; small amounts of the indanyl ester were present during the first two hours following each dose. Only trace amounts of benzyl penicillin were observed. The concentrations of carbenicillin in urine were very high, and in many subjects exceeded 1000 mcg/ml. The increased dosage from 500 mg four times a day to 1000 mg four times a day for the carbenicillin ester gave a marked increase in carbenicillin content of serum, but a similar change was not observed for the serum ester content. This implies that only a small percentage of the total dose of the carbenicillin ester escaped into the circulatory system.

At the highest dosage regimen (1000 mg four times a day) for the indanyl ester there appeared to be a slight increase in peak levels after the first nine to ten doses. This was not so apparent at the lower dosage regimen (500 mg four times a day), It was also noted that the antibiotic serum titers were prolonged after dosage at night.

Table 9 highlights this essential difference between the multiple dose regimens of these antibiotics.

Summary

Carbenicillin indanyl sodium is a new semisynthetic penicillin. It is an orally effective derivative of carbenicillin. The indanyl carbenicillin is acid-stable and rapidly absorbed from the gastrointestinal tract and is hydrolyzed *in vivo* to produce carbenicillin and metabolic by-products derived from indanol. Orally administered carbenicillin indanyl sodium provides the same therapeutic effect as parenterally administered carbenicillin disodium in experimental infections in mice and rats. The serum and urine levels of carbenicillin produced by a single 1.0 gram oral dose of carbenicillin indanyl sodium in man compare favorably with those following a single intramuscular injection of 1.0 gram of carbenicillin. The urinary concentrations of carbenicillin achieved by a multiple dosage regimen of indanyl carbenicillin sodium (.5 gram four times a day) in man easily exceed the MIC values of common urinary tract pathogens.

REFERENCES

1. Batson HC: An Introduction to Statistics in the Medical Sciences. Minneapolis, Minnesota, Burgess Publishing Co., 1956.
2. English AA, McBride TJ, Conover LH, et al: 3-Substituted nitrofurantoins as urinary-tract anti-infectives. Antimicrobial Agents and Chemotherapy, 434-444, 1966.

TREATMENT OF URINARY TRACT INFECTIONS WITH OXOLINIC ACID

In Patients with Normal and Impaired Renal Function

• Oxolinic acid was well tolerated in this group of patients with chronic urinary tract infection. This drug was efficient in eradication of susceptible organisms from the urine, but the frequent development of resistance is a major concern.

K. MOHRING, M.D.
PAUL O. MADSEN, M.D.

Oxolinic acid is being investigated in search for new and more effective agents in the treatment of urinary tract infections. Its structure (Fig. 1) and antibacterial spectrum are very similar to those of nalidixic acid. The minimal inhibitory concentration for common gram-negative organisms found in urinary tract infections, however, is much lower (1/5 to 1/10) than that of nalidixic acid, being about 1-6 mcg/ml.[1,2] We have investigated the efficacy and safety of oxolinic acid in the treatment of chronic urinary tract infections in patients with normal and reduced kidney function.

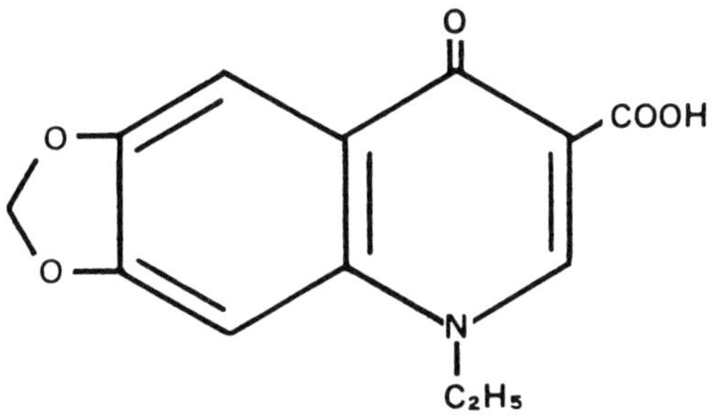

Materials and Methods

Male patients, practically all with chronic urinary tract infection, were included in the study. Most of the patients had normal renal function; nineteen had reduced renal function. The patients' average age was approximately 70 years. Almost all the urinary tract infections were associated with lower urinary tract disease, such as benign hypertrophy of the prostate, cancer of the prostate, bladder stones, and bladder tumors. Most of the patients with impaired renal function had indwelling catheters. This patient group represents a very chronic and persistent type of urinary tract infection. Most patients had been treated previously with other chemotherapeutic agents or antibiotics, and thus

Figure 1.

Oxolinic Acid: 5-ethyl-5, 8-dihydro-8-oxo-1, 3-dioxolo (4,5-g)-quinoline-7-carboxylic acid. Molecular weight: 261.2 Empirical formula: $NO_5C_{13}H_{11}$.

many of the cases represented recurrent or persistent infections. Urine cultures were obtained from midstream urine, and counts higher than 5000 colonies/ml were considered positive although the great majority of the patients had counts higher than 100,000 colonies/ml. The usual dosage of oxolinic acid was 750 mg twice daily. In order to evaluate possible accumulation of oxolinic acid during treatment, determinations of serum concentration of biologically active oxolinic acid were carried out on blood samples obtained two hours following the last oral administration on the first, seventh, fourteenth and twenty-first day of treatment in both patient groups. Determinations of urine concentration of biologically active oxolinic acid were carried out

Dr. Mohring is Resident in Urology, Veterans Administration Hospital, Madison, Wisconsin and Dr. Madsen is Associate Professor of Urology, University of Wisconsin and Chief of Urology, Veterans Administration Hospital, Madison, Wisconsin.

TABLE 1

Bacteriological response of 98 gram-negative sensitive microorganisms sensitive to oxolinic acid during treatment with oxolinic acid 750 mg q 12 h for 10-15 days. Sensitivity is defined as a zone of 15 mm or more around a 5 μg disc.

Infecting microorganism (sens. to oxolinic acid)	No. of strains	Eradicated during treatment	Persisted during treatment (developed resistance)
E. coli	44	89%	11%
Proteus	30	67%	33%
Klebsiella	24	79%	21%

on 24-hour urine specimens collected on the same treatment days. A two-fold tube dilution technique was used with a sensitive *E. coli* strain as test organism. Sensitivity testing was carried out with various disc concentrations (from 0.5 to 5 mcg). Additional laboratory work-up included complete blood count, SGOT, and alkaline phosphatases done before and at the end of treatment.

Results

The bacteriological and clinical response of the treatment is illustrated in Tables 1-3. The results of the bioassays are illustrated in Figures 2 and 3 and listed in detail in Table 3. The serum concentrations of oxolinic acid obtained at intervals from one to twelve hours following the administration of 750 mg twice daily in eight patients with normal renal function reached peak levels after two hours, averaging 0.9 mcg/ml on the first day of treatment, 1.9 mcg/ml on the seventh and 2.1 mcg/ml on the fourteenth day of treatment. These very low serum concentrations indicate that oxolinic acid should not be used in the treatment of systemic infections where high serum and tissue concentrations are desirable, but should

be used only in urinary tract infections, similar to the use of nalidixic acid and nitrofurantoin.

The serum concentrations following administration of 750 mg twice daily of oxolinic acid to 19 patients with impaired renal function were only slightly higher than those in patients with normal renal function (Figure 3). Neither group shows a tendency to accumulation of biologically active substance in the serum over a treatment period of 21 days. The mean 24-hour urine concentration in eight patients with normal renal function averaged from 44 to 96 mcg/ml, a concentration which must be considered therapeutically adequate since it is many times higher than the minimal inhibitory concentration for most common infecting organisms in the urinary tract. Also in the patients with impaired renal function even the first day average urine concentrations were high (Table 3), which demonstrates that the bacteriological response in these azotemic patients was as good as in patients with normal renal function. The total amount of recovered oxolinic acid in the 24-hour urine of patients with normal renal function averaged

Time of evaluation	Results		
	Neg. culture	Reinfection	Persistence
Last day of treatment (93 patients)	47%	29%	24%
1-6 Weeks following treatment (83 patients)	41%		59%

TABLE 2

Bacteriological response in 93 patients infected with one or more organisms sensitive to oxolinic acid and treated with oxolinic acid 750 mg q 12 h for 10-15 days. Colony counts less than 5,000 colonies/ml are considered negative.

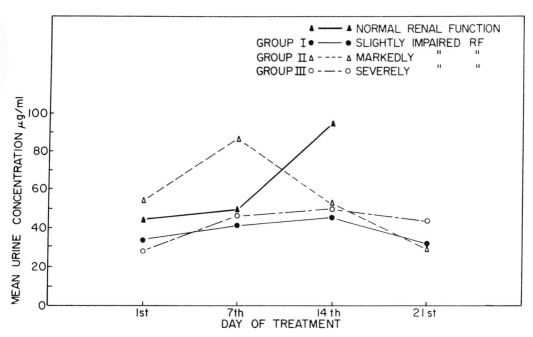

Figure 2. Mean urine concentrations (μg/ml) during 14-21 days of treatment with oxolinic acid 750 mg every 12 hours in patients with normal renal function and with varying degrees of impairment of renal function. There is a sufficiently high urine concentration of oxolinic acid for therapeutical purposes in all four groups of patients.

For definition of renal function impairment see Table 3.

6.5 per cent, ranging from 1.8-21.2 per cent. In patients with impaired renal function, the average excretion was also 6.5 per cent, ranging from 0.9-42 per cent. It therefore appears that even patients with poor renal function do not need an initial loading dose in order to achieve immediate and effective urine concentrations.

In the patients with normal kidney function 79 per cent of the organisms found sensitive by the disc sensitivity method were eradicated during the treatment, whereas two per cent persisted despite sensitivity according to the disc sensitivity test and 19 per cent developed resistance during the treatment. In patients with impaired renal function, eleven organisms were sensitive *in vitro* and nine of the eleven were eliminated during therapy. Resistance as a rule had developed within one to three days of treatment. This frequent development of resistance has also been found following the administration of nalidixic acid.[1]

In a comparative randomized study of 60 patients with gram-negative urinary tract infections where 30 patients were treated with nalidixic acid, 1 gm four times daily, and 30 patients with oxolinic acid, 1 gm twice daily, for 14 days, the bacteriological results of the two groups were not significantly different. In both groups a negative urine culture, which remained negative for one to two weeks following the treatment, was accomplished in 40 per cent of the patients.

The most common side effects of therapy were nausea, vertigo, insomnia and drowsiness. There was no overall evidence of a toxic effect on the renal function in the normal or in the azotemic patients. Other laboratory tests conducted before and after treatment indicated no toxic effect on liver function and hematopoietic function. The number of side effects previously mentioned was not significantly

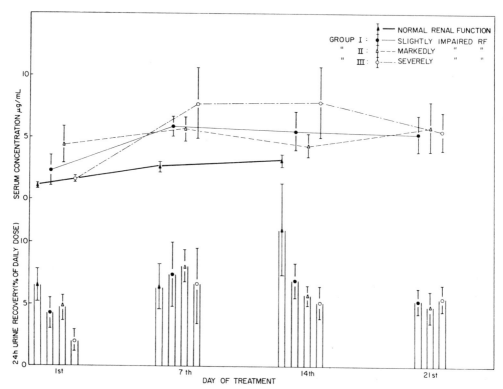

Figure 3. Mean serum concentrations (μg/ml $\pm$ 1 standard error) of oxolinic acid and recovery rate of oxolinic acid over a 24-hour period in patients with normal and varying degrees of impairment of renal function. There is no significant difference in the serum values of biologically active substance on the various days of determination, and there is no significant difference in the 24-hour urine recovery of biologically active substance in the four groups of patients. For definition of renal function impairment see Table 3.

different from that found in patients with normal renal function.[3]

Discussion

The effect of oxolinic acid has been found very similar to that of nalidixic acid. The advantage of oxolinic acid over nalidixic acid would be in the somewhat more prolonged effect of the oxolinic acid since adequate urine concentrations are found up to 12 hours following a single dose. Since we found no difference in the efficacy of the various dosages of oxolinic acid tested, we recommend a dosage of 750 mg twice daily. Patients should only be treated if disc sensitivity indicates that the microorganism is sensitive. If the treatment

has not resulted in a negative urine within 48 to 72 hours, the treatment can probably be considered a failure since the infecting organism has by then developed resistance to the oxolinic acid.

The possibility that biologically inactive metabolic products of oxolinic acid, most likely inactivated as the glucuronide,[3,4] can accumulate and be toxic to patients with impaired renal function can be excluded by our study.

Summary

A new chemotherapeutic agent, oxolinic acid, was tested in the treatment of chronic urinary tract infections in patients with nor-

TABLE 3

Mean urine concentration (mcg/ml) and bacteriological response during 21 days of treatment with oxolinic acid, 750 mg q 12 h.

		Group I	Group II	Group III
No. of Patients		8	7	4
	[a]BUN	25.9 ± 9.96	30.4 ± 6.95	64.5 ± 7.14
Day of treatment	[b]S.C.	1.65 ± 0.29	2.3 ± 0.23	4.4 ± 1.12
	[c]C.C.	53.4 ± 12.5	31.7 ± 5.40	16 ± 2.94
1st		34.1	54.5	28
(range)		8.7-64	14-155.6	18-34
7th		42.2	87.8	46.0
(range)		11.4-155.5	14.8-155.6	2-97.9
14th		46.4	53.4	50.5
(range)		18.2-102	16.7-113.6	16-70
21st		32.4	31.3	44.1
(range)		19.3-46.2	13.6-64	19-71.4
No. of sensitive organisms		5	4	2
No. eradicated during treatment		4	4	2

[a]Blood Urea Nitrogen   (Mean ± 1 standard deviation)
[b]Serum Creatinine   (Mean ± 1 standard deviation)
[c]Creatinine Clearance   (Mean ± 1 standard deviation)

Group I: Slightly impaired renal function
Group II: Markedly impaired renal function
Group III: Severely impaired renal function

mal and impaired renal function. The drug was well tolerated in both groups. Oral administration of 750 mg twice daily resulted in sufficiently high urine concentrations in both groups. The drug was found to be safe and efficient and showed no accumulation in the blood, but produced high urine concentrations even in patients with poor renal function. In patients with normal renal function it eliminated from the urine 79 per cent of gram-negative microorganisms sensitive to oxolinic acid and cured 41 per cent of the infections. In patients with impaired renal function, nine of eleven sensitive microorganisms were

eradicated during treatment. The high incidence of reinfection in this group was mainly due to resistant enterococci. The low serum concentrations and high urine concentrations limit the usefulness of this drug to urinary tract infections due to susceptible gram-negative organisms. The frequent development of resistance is a major concern.

REFERENCES

1. Atlas E. Clark H, Silverblatt F, et al: Nalidixic acid and oxolinic acid in the treatment of chronic bacteriuria. Ann Int Med 70:713, 1969.
2. Data on file at Warner-Lambert Research Institute, Morris Plains, N.J.
3. Madsen PO and Rhodes PR: Oxolinic acid, a new chemotherapeutic agent in the treatment of urinary tract infections. Journ Urol. In Print.
4. Stamey TA, Nemoy NJ and Higgins M: The clinical use of nalidixic acid. Invest Urol 6:582, 1969.

Never forget that it is not a pneumonia, but a pneumonic man who is your patient. Not a typhoid fever, but a typhoid man.
Sir William Withey Gull (1816-1890) *Published Writings* (ed. by T. D. Acland),
Memoir II.

CLINICAL EXPERIENCE WITH ORAL CARBENICILLIN

• The oral formulation of carbenicillin appears
to be an effective agent in the treatment of acute
and chronic urinary tract infections. When available for general use this preparation may be
valuable in the treatment of selected patients.

WILLIAM A. TAYLOR, M.D.
WILLIAM J. HOLLOWAY, M.D.

Carbenicillin, a semi-synthetic penicillin, has a wide spectrum of activity against gram-negative and gram-positive bacteria.[1] Particularly significant to the clinician is the bactericidal effect of this new antibiotic against strains of *Pseudomonas aeruginosa* and *Proteus* species. The parenteral formulation of carbenicillin has now been used extensively in the treatment of patients with infections due to gram-negative bacilli.[2-4] The current formulation of carbenicillin can not be given by the oral route because it is rapidly inactivated by gastric acid. Recently, an indanyl ester of carbenicillin has been made available which is well absorbed when given by the oral route and has essentially the same antibacterial activity as the parent compound.[5] This ester is metabolized into carbenicillin upon absorption into the blood stream and is excreted into the urinary tract as carbenicillin. Preliminary studies carried out in our laboratory indicate that the blood level of carbenicillin following oral dosing with 500 mg of the indanyl ester is extremely variable ranging from less than 2 mcg/ml to 4.5 mcg/ml. In the same volunteers, urinary levels of carbenicillin following this dose of the indanyl ester are more consistent, ranging from 400 to 500 mcg/ml in aliquots of urine collected two to three hours after dosing. The broad antibac-

terial spectrum of carbenicillin and its indanyl ester, coupled with the consistent urinary levels of antibiotic obtained after oral administration, prompted a clinical trial of this formulation in the treatment of patients with acute and chronic urinary tract infection.

Material and Methods

Sixty-three patients were selected for inclusion in this study. These patients were from the Medical and Surgical Services of the Wilmington Medical Center, the Pyelonephritis Clinic of the Wilmington Medical Center and private outpatients at the Brandywine Medical Center. Of the total of sixty-three patients treated, forty-six were females and seventeen males. They were classified as follows: 18 patients, acute cystitis; 3 patients, chronic cystitis; 13 patients, acute pyelonephritis; and 29 patients, chronic pyelonephritis. This clinical categorization of patients was based upon history, symptomatology (fever, loin pain, rigor, dysuria, frequency), the results of laboratory evaluation and in some instances intravenous pyelogram.

Urine cultures were obtained by clean-caught midstream technique or by urethral catheterization. Occasional cultures were obtained by suprapubic bladder aspiration technique. Standard microbiologic techniques were used with a 0.01 ml wire loop; a colony

Dr. Taylor is Chief Resident in Medicine and Dr. Holloway is
Director, Infectious Disease Research Laboratory, Wilmington Medical Center, Wilmington, Delaware.

173

count greater than 10^5 was considered evidence of significant infection. Speciation of the organisms was carried out by the standard techniques. Susceptibility of pathogens isolated was determined using a disc-agar diffusion technique with 100 mcg discs of carbenicillin.

The indanyl ester of carbenicillin was supplied as a tablet containing 500 mg by the research laboratories of Pfizer Company. The usual dose schedule was 500 mg of oral carbenicillin every six hours for a minimum period of ten days to two weeks. Modification of this treatment program was necessary in a few patients in whom long-term suppressive therapy with carbenicillin was necessary to maintain a sterile urine. In addition, in a few instances, the dose of carbenicillin was increased to 1000 mg or 1500 mg every six hours in an attempt to sterilize the urine in patients with chronic bacteriuria.

Repeat urine cultures were obtained during therapy and following therapy in all instances for at least a minimum of six weeks.

Pre- and post-treatment toxicity studies included hemogram, chemistry 12 profile and urinalysis. Carbenicillin serum and urine levels were obtained at representative intervals in a large number of the patients in this study.

Results

Forty-two of the sixty-three patients in this study experienced a satisfactory result from therapy while there were eighteen failures and three patients categorized as qualified successes. The overwhelming majority of the failures occurred in patients with chronic pyelonephritis.

Cystitis: Seventeen of the eighteen patients with acute cystitis were treated with a successful outcome. The one patient with acute cystitis who failed to respond to carbenicillin therapy had a persistent infection with *Escherichia coli* with no change in the antibiotic susceptibility pattern of this organism following therapy. Included in the seventeen successful outcomes were eleven patients infected with *Escherichia coli* and one whose infection was due to *Pseudomonas aeruginosa*.

All three patients with chronic cystitis due to *Escherichia coli* experienced a successful result with treatment with oral carbenicillin.

Pyelonephritis: Thirteen patients in this study were categorized as having acute pyelonephritis, and all thirteen of these patients responded to a course of oral carbenicillin therapy. The pathogen in each of these thirteen cases was as follows: *Escherichia coli* = six patients; *Proteus mirabilis* = three patients; beta-hemolytic streptococcus = two patients; and enterococcus = two patients.

Twenty-nine patients with chronic pyelonephritis were included in this study with the majority of these patients having obstructive uropathy and abnormal intravenous urograms. In nine instances, patients with chronic pyelonephritis had an unqualified successful outcome resulting from a course of oral carbenicillin therapy ranging from two to four weeks. Three patients with chronic pyelonephritis were considered as having qualified successful outcomes from the oral carbenicillin therapy. These patients have been classified as having qualified successes because on long-term suppressive therapy with carbenicillin in a dosage of 1 gm four times a day, they have been kept free of bacteriuria and had no clinical relapses. Two of these three patients with chronic *Pseudomonas* pyelonephritis have failed to respond to therapy with any other antibiotic regimen in the past.

Seventeen of the twenty-nine patients in the chronic pyelonephritis group failed to respond to therapy with oral carbenicillin and are detailed as follows: five of eight patients with chronic *Escherichia coli* pyelonephritis failed to respond to oral carbenicillin therapy. In two of these five patients who failed to respond, the *Escherichia coli* isolated on the original urine culture was resistant to carbenicillin. Two additional patients who had a susceptible strain of *Escherichia coli* at the onset of treatment with carbenicillin acquired resistant strains of *Klebsiella* species. The fifth patient with *Escherichia coli* infection who failed to respond maintained a susceptible strain of *Escherichia coli* in his urine. However, there was no clinical or bacteriologic improvement.

In one patient of three who had chronic *Proteus mirabilis*, the organism was replaced with a resistant strain of *Pseudomonas aeruginosa*. One patient with chronic pyelonephritis due to an *Enterobacter* species failed to respond to therapy even though the original infecting organism was sensitive to carbenicillin; it was replaced with a carbenicillin resistant *Enterobacter*. Two of three patients with mixed infections causing chronic pyelonephritis failed to respond to therapy with carbenicillin, in each instance the susceptible pathogens being replaced with resistant *Klebsiella*.

Eight patients with chronic *Pseudomonas* pyelonephritis failed to respond to therapy with oral carbenicillin. In four of these cases, the original susceptible *Pseudomonas* was eradicated but replaced with resistant organisms (*Escherichia coli* in two instances and *Klebsiella* species in two instances). In two patients, urine culture revealed a *Pseudomonas aeruginosa* still sensitive to carbenicillin with the same pyocine typing as the organism isolated prior to therapy. In two additional failures the *Pseudomonas aeruginosa* had been susceptible to carbenicillin prior to therapy, but became resistant during the course of therapy although the pyocine type again remained the same.

Side Effects

There were a minimal number of side effects during therapy in the sixty-three patients in this study. Gastrointestinal distress (nausea and dyspepsia) occurred in five subjects but required termination of therapy in only one instance. One patient was seen who experienced transient dermatographia while receiving oral carbenicillin, and it was thought that this was probably causally related to the antibiotic therapy. There were four instances in which mild hematologic abnormalities were noted during the course of therapy. In two patients, there was mild leukopenia (total white blood count of less than 4,000), and in the other two patients there was an eosinophilia of greater than 10%. In all four instances of hematologic abnormality oral carbenicillin therapy was continued, and the abnormal value reverted to normal.

Antibiotic Levels

Serum specimens were obtained from patients on multiple doses of oral carbenicillin at two, three and four hours following ingestion of a 500 mg dose with considerable variation in the measured levels of carbenicillin. The sensitivity of the technique used did not measure levels below 2 mcg/ml, and in more than 50% of the patients tested, the levels at two-, three-, and four-hour intervals fell below this level. In the remaining fourteen patients, the levels ranged from 2 to 5 mcg/ml. In a representative number of cases, the dosage of carbenicillin was increased to 1 and 1.5 gm of carbenicillin taken at six-hour intervals. Slightly higher serum levels of carbenicillin occurred in these patients on increased dosage with the serum carbenicillin level ranging from 3 to 6 mcg/ml two hours following the 1 gm dose of oral carbenicillin and ranging from 5 to 8 mcg/ml one hour following a 1.5 gm oral dose of carbenicillin.

Likewise, the urine levels in these patients showed considerable variation. Random urine levels obtained in patients attending pyelonephritis clinic (usually three to four hours following a dose of carbenicillin) gave levels ranging from 200 mcg/ml to 1600 mcg/ml. The mean carbenicillin levels for eighteen patients receiving 500 mg orally every six hours was 575 mg/ml.

Summary

The indanyl ester of carbenicillin administered by the oral route appears to be a well-tolerated, effective agent in the treatment of acute urinary tract infections. Further investigation will be necessary to determine the proper role of this antibiotic in the treatment of patients with chronic pyelonephritis. In our experience, there are selected patients with chronic *Pseudomonas* urinary tract infection in which the indanyl ester of carbenicillin appears to be the oral antibiotic of choice.

REFERENCES

1. Brumfitt W, Percival A and Leigh DA: Clinical laboratory studies with carbenicillin. Lancet 1:1289-1293, 1967.
2. Taylor WA and Holloway WJ: Carbenicillin in the treatment of the critically ill patient. In press.
3. Labowitz R and Holloway WJ: Carbenicillin in the treatment of severe infections. Curr Ther Res 11:143-149, 1969.
4. Hoffman TA and Bullock WE: Carbenicillin therapy of pseudomonas and other gram-negative bacillary infections. Am Int Med 73:165-172, 1970.
5. Informational Brochure on CP-15,464 (oral carbenicillin). Pfizer Laboratories, Groton, Conn.

CEPHAPIRIN: Clinical, Pharmacological, and Microbiological Studies

SIMON JAMESON, M.D.
MARTIN C. McHENRY, M.D.
RAY A. VANOMMEN, M.D.
THOMAS L. GAVAN, M.D.
DONALD G. VIDT, M.D.
DIANE A. BUTLER, B.S.

Cephapirin [sodium 7-(pyrid-4-yl-thio ace-tamido) cephalosporanate] is a new semisynthetic derivative of 7- aminocephalosporonic acid which appears to have an antibacterial spectrum similar to cephalothin and cephaloridine.[1-2] Cephapirin is not significantly absorbed by the oral route and requires parenteral injection.[3] It seems to cause less pain and, after intravenous or intramuscular administration, is better tolerated than cephalothin; unlike cephaloridine it does not appear to be nephrotoxic. Because of these advantages, further study of the drug seemed to be indicated.

The present study was undertaken to determine the following: (1) *in vitro* susceptibility of clinical isolates of gram-positive cocci and gram-negative bacilli to cephapirin, (2) the serum half-life of cephapirin after a 1 gm intravenous dose in persons with normal renal function, and (3) the efficacy and safety of cephapirin in patients with infections due to susceptible organisms.

Materials and Methods

Cephapirin sodium (BL-P1322) was supplied as a sterile powder in vials containing 0.5 or 1.0 gm for intramuscular or intravenous use. Cephapirin in powder form (Lot # 70 F241 - Potency 975 μg/mg) was supplied for use in the tests of bacterial susceptibility.

Two hundred ninety strains of gram-negative bacilli and gram-positive cocci isolated from patients at the Cleveland Clinic during March 1971 were studied. Organisms were

The authors are with the Department of Internal Medicine, Section of Infectious Diseases; the Department of Microbiology; and the Department of Hypertension and Nephrology, the Cleveland Clinic Foundation, Cleveland, Ohio.

identified according to routine bacteriologic methods.[4] These included 64 strains of *Proteus mirabilis*, 48 of *Klebsiella*, 31 of *E. coli*, 20 of *Enterobacter*, 19 of *Pseudomonas aeruginosa*, 36 of *Staphylococcus aureus*, 30 of *Staphylococcus epidermidis*, 30 of enterococcus group, 7 of alpha hemolytic streptococci, 11 of group A beta hemolytic streptococci, and 3 of *Diplococcus pneumoniae*.

The minimum inhibitory concentration (MIC) of cephapirin for 182 strains of gram-negative bacilli and 96 strains of gram-positive cocci was determined by a microdilution technique.[5] Transparent plastic wells containing the antibiotic in concentrations ranging from 0.2 to 200 μg/ml in brain-heart infusion broth (BBL) were inoculated with 0.05 ml of a 1:1000 dilution of an overnight broth culture. The final concentration of cephapirin ranged from 0.1 to 100 μg/ml. The minimum inhibitory concentration (MIC) was read as the lowest concentration of cephapirin which produced complete inhibition of growth after overnight incubation at 35 C.

The MIC of cephapirin for 11 strains of group A beta hemolytic streptococci, 7 strains of alpha hemolytic streptococci, and 3 strains of *Diplococcus pneumoniae* was determined by a twofold macrodilution method because end point determinations by the microdilution method were difficult with those organisms. The same cephapirin dilution schedule, innoculum ratio, and end point evaluation were used with both methods. Susceptibility of the 290 bacterial isolates was also determined by the agar disc diffusion method using a 30 μg cephapirin disc according to the standardized technique of Bauer and associates.[6]

Organisms	Number of Strains	BHIB* (μg/ml)	N.B.** (μg/ml)	TSB‡ with dextrose (μg/ml)	TSB‡ without dextrose (μg/ml)
Klebsiella	10	22	15	12	21
E. coli					
Proteus Mirabilis	10	24	10	24	16
Proteus mirabilis	15	18	2.1	16	36

*Brain-heart infusion broth (B.B.L.).
**Nutrient broth (B.B.L.).
‡Trypticase soy broth (B.B.L.).

TABLE 1

Geometric Mean M I C
of Cephapirin with Different
Broth Culture Media

In order to determine the influence of different culture media on the MIC of cephapirin, 10 strains of *Klebsiella*, 10 of *E. coli*, and 15 of *Proteus mirabilis* were tested simultaneously by the microdilution method employing four different broth media. Overnight cultures and serial dilutions of cephapirin were prepared in brain-heart infusion broth (BBL), nutrient broth (BBL), Trypticase soy broth with dextrose (BBL), and Trypticase soy broth without dextrose (BBL). The MIC's were read as described after 18-hour incubation at 35 C. The geometric mean MIC for those strains was determined for each of the four media. The paired T test was applied to evaluate the significance of any observed differences.

Seven adult volunteers with normal renal function (endogenous creatinine clearances > 80 ml/min/1.73 m² body surface area) were selected for study after informed consent was obtained. A 1 gm dose of cephapirin diluted in 25 to 50 ml of normal saline was administered intravenously to each person during a period ranging from 2 to 12 minutes. Venous blood was drawn prior to the infusion and at intervals of 15 min., ½, 1, 2, 3 and 6 hours after the infusion. The venous blood was allowed to clot, and serum was collected, frozen, and shipped promptly to the Bristol Laboratories, Syracuse, New York. Assays of the concentration of cephapirin in the serum were performed promptly in the Bristol Labora-

tories by an agar-plate bioassay method using *Sarcina lutea* ATC 9341 as the test organism.

Values of serum concentration versus time plotted on a semilogarithmic graph showed a linear decline of cephapirin beginning 15 minutes after the intravenous injection. Linear regression lines were calculated by the method of least squares; the slope of each line was used to calculate the serum half-life of cephapirin.

Twenty-nine patients hospitalized in the Cleveland Clinic Hospital from June 1970 to March 1971 were treated with cephapirin for a variety of infections. Informed consent was obtained from each patient or from his responsible relatives. There were 17 males and 12 females, whose ages ranged from 17 to 76 years. Except in one instance, no other antibiotics were given simultaneously. The criterion for selection for treatment with cephapirin was the presence of an infection presumed or proved to be due to an organism susceptible to this drug. Ten of the twenty-nine patients had histories of allergy to the penicillins.

Cephapirin was given intramuscularly or intravenously in individual doses ranging from 0.5 to 2.0 gm at intervals of every 4 to 12 hours. In patients with severely impaired renal function, the drug was usually given at intervals of 8 to 12 hours. The duration of cephapirin therapy ranged from 3 to 48 days

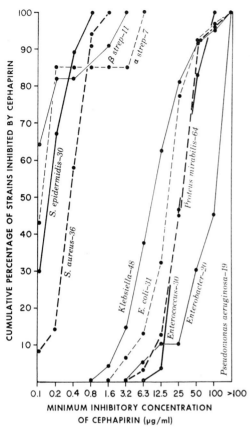

Figure 1: Graphic representation of the cumulative percentage of the various isolates susceptible to increasing concentrations of cephapirin.

and averaged 16.1 days for the entire group. The total dosage of cephapirin ranged from 6 to 516 gm with an average of 113.9 gm for the entire group.

We examined each of the 29 patients daily. Appropriate measures to control underlying diseases and to treat any complications were employed as indicated. Cultures of sites of infection were obtained before, during, and after therapy. The susceptibility of all pathogens was determined by the agar-disc diffusion method or the microdilution method, or both. Laboratory studies including complete blood cell counts, urinalysis, and determinations of serum glutamic oxaloacetic transaminase, lactic dehydrogenase, bilirubin, alkaline phosphatase, blood urea nitrogen, and serum creatinine were carried out before, during, and after therapy.

The results of treatment with cephapirin were classified in four categories: (1) Successful—disappearance of all signs and symptoms of acute infection with sterile cultures during and after therapy. (2) Qualified success— disappearance of all signs and symptoms of acute infection, except for one of the following conditions: cultures of the urine or sputum or other extravascular sites of infection continued to be positive during therapy; bacteriologic or clinical relapse occurred after discontinuation of therapy; or post-treatment cultures were not obtained for various reasons.

SUB-JECT	TIME AFTER 1 GRAM I.V. DOSE OF CEPHAPIRIN SODIUM, HOURS							SERUM HALF-LIFE HRS.
	0.25	0.5	1	2	3	4	6	
#1	50	22	12	3.5	2	—	0.3	0.83
#2	37	14	4.4	1.3	0.5	—	<0.1	0.47
#3	20	8.3	2.8	0.8	0.2	—	<0.1	0.44
#4	46	26	12	4.6	3.2	—	0.6	0.97
#5	34	14	5.6	—	0.8	0.4	<0.1	0.62
#6	48	20	9.3	2.4	0.5	—	<0.1	0.44
#7	22	10	3.3	2.8	0.4	0.2	<0.1	0.54
MEAN							0.615 ± 0.2 S.D.	

*Endogenous creatinine clearance >80 ml/min/1.73m^2 body surface area.

TABLE 2

Serum Levels of Cephapirin in 7 Subjects with Normal Renal Function*

TABLE 3

RESULTS OF CEPHAPIRIN THERAPY IN 10 PATIENTS WITH 12 EPISODES OF
NONBACTEREMIC URINARY TRACT INFECTIONS

Infection	Causative Organism(s) (M I C of cephapirin, μg/ml)	Results of Therapy
Acute pyelonephritis	*E. coli* (12.5)	Successful
	E. coli (>100)	Successful
	Proteus mirabilis (50)	Successful
	Klebsiella sp (50)+	Qualified success (relapse after Rx)
	E. coli (100)	Qualified success (relapse after Rx)
	*E. coli**	Qualified success (persistence of bacteriuria despite symptomatic improvement)
	*E. coli**	Unsuccessful (Pseudomonas superinfection)
	E. coli and *Klebsiella sp*	Unsuccessful (Pseudomonas superinfection)
Acute cystitis	*E. coli* and *Proteus mirabilis* (25)	Qualified success (relapse after Rx)
	Proteus morgani (25)	Indeterminate
Chronic pyelonephritis	*Proteus mirabilis* (25)	Indeterminate
	Klebsiella sp (>100)**	Indeterminate

*Two episodes in this patient.   **Two episodes in this patient.

(3) Unsuccessful—failure to eradicate acute infection or development of significant superinfection. (4) Indeterminate — intervening antibiotic therapy prevented evaluation of effects of cephapirin therapy.

Results

The cumulative percentage of the various isolates susceptible to increasing concentrations of cephapirin is shown in Figure 1. One hundred percent of gram-positive cocci, except enterococci, were inhibited by 6.3 μg/ml or less of cephapirin. Gram-negative bacilli and enterococci showed less susceptibility to the drug.

Differences in the geometric mean MIC's of cephapirin for strains of *E. coli*, *Klebsiella* and *Proteus mirabilis* tested in different broth media by the microdilution method are shown in Table 1. The geometric mean MIC of

cephapirin in nutrient broth was significantly lower for *E. coli* (p<0.01) and *Proteus mirabilis* (p<0.001) than when those strains were tested in other media.

Pertinent data from each of the seven subjects studied after a single intravenous dose of 1.0 gm of cephapirin are listed in Table 2. Peak serum concentrations of cephapirin were present 15 minutes after the injection and averaged 36.7 μg/ml for the group. Cephapirin concentrations declined rapidly to negligible levels at six hours. The serum half-life of cephapirin ranged from 0.4 to 0.8 hr. with a mean of about 0.6 hr. Our preliminary unpublished data indicate that the serum half-life of cephapirin was somewhat prolonged in patients with severely impaired renal function.

Ten patients with 12 episodes of urinary tract infection were treated. (Table 3) Five

Infection	Causative Organisms(s) (M I C of cephapirin, μg/ml)	Result of Treatment
Lung abscess	*Klebsiella sp* (1.6) and *Proteus mirabilis* (12.5)	Successful
Pneumonia	*Klebsiella sp* (6.3)	Unsuccessful
	Klebsiella sp (1.6)	Successful*
	Klebsiella sp (1.6) and *Enterobacter sp* (12.5)	Indeterminate (intervening gentamicin therapy)
	Proteus mirabilis (12.5)	Successful
	Staphylococcus aureus (0.8)	Unsuccessful
Acute purulent bronchitis	*Diplococcus pneumoniae* (sensitive by disc method)	Successful
	Staphylococcus aureus (0.4)	Successful

*Pneumonia cleared before therapy had to be stopped because of bullous erythema multiforme; the latter condition was successfully treated with adrenal glucocorticoids.

TABLE 4

Results of Cephapirin Therapy In 8 Patients with Acute Respiratory Infections

of those patients had renal transplants, five had impaired renal function, one had a neurogenic bladder. *E. coli, Klebsiella* or *Proteus* were the causative organisms. The MIC of cephapirin for the various pathogens was determined in nine instances and ranged from 12.5 to more than 100 μg/ml. In three patients, long-term oral antibacterial therapy was started before post-treatment urine cultures were obtained; although the urine cultures were sterile during cephapirin therapy, the results of treatment were classified as indeterminate. Treatment was unsuccessful in only two patients; both had severely malfunctioning renal transplants which later required nephrectomy.

Eight patients received cephapirin therapy for severe respiratory infections—pneumonia, lung abscess, or acute purulent bronchitis caused by various gram-positive cocci or gram-negative bacilli. (Table 4) Isolates were tested by the microdilution method in seven of the eight patients—all of the strains tested had an MIC of 12.5 μg/ml or less of cephapirin. Treatment was clearly unsuccessful in only two patients. One of the two patients had failed to respond to other antibacterial

drugs and was in the late stages of necrotizing aspiration pneumonia when cephapirin treatment was begun. The other patient had a renal transplant, intensive immunosuppressive therapy, and fulminating staphylococcal pneumonia which failed to respond to other antibiotics after cephapirin treatment was discontinued.

The results of cephapirin therapy of bacteremic infections are shown in Table 5. Three patients with uncomplicated bacteremia and four patients with bacterial endocarditis were treated. Of the three patients with uncomplicated bacteremia, therapy was successful in two and a qualified success in one. In the latter patient, staphylococcal bacteremia cleared during therapy, but the underlying liver abscess persisted. Of the four patients with bacterial endocarditis, one with a resistant strain of *E. coli* had persistent bacteremia despite cephapirin therapy; bloodstream infection was controlled by another drug. One patient received other antibiotics for more than one day prior to cephapirin; another received an alternative antibiotic when cephapirin had to be discontinued because of drug fever; results of cephapirin therapy in those two patients with

Infection	Causative Organism (MIC of cephapirin, μg/ml)	Result of Treatment
Bacteremia	*E. coli* (12.5)	Successful
	Staphylococcus aureus (0.8)	Qualified success
	Klebsiella sp (12.5)	Successful
Bacterial endocarditis	*Staphylococcus aureus* (0.1)	
	Staphylococcus epidermitis (0.1)	Indeterminate
	Corynebacterium pyogenes (0.1)	Indeterminate
	E. coli (50)	Unsuccessful

TABLE 5

Results of Cephapirin Therapy of Bacteremic Infections in 7 Patients

endocarditis were classified as indeterminate. The fourth patient had staphylococcal endocarditis, which was cured after 43 days of intravenous cephapirin therapy.

In four patients, miscellaneous infections, including wound infections, chronic draining osteomyelitis, and staphylococcal pyoarthrosis, (Table 6), responded favorably to cephapirin and appropriate surgical drainage.

The overall clinical results in 31 episodes of infection were as follows: successful, 11; a qualified success, 9; unsuccessful, 5; and indeterminate, 6. If the categories of successful and qualified success are combined, and if the indeterminate cases are excluded, the overall rate of success of cephapirin therapy was 80 percent (20/25) and the failure rate was 20 percent (5/25).

The number and types of adverse reactions to cephapirin are listed in Table 7. Side effects occurred in about one-third of our patients. In general, they were mild and of no clinical significance. However, in three patients, severe side effects necessitated termination of cephapirin therapy; those included bullous erythema multiforme, drug fever with transient leukopenia, and generalized maculopapular rash with eosinophilia. There was no evidence of nephrotoxicity; thrombophlebitis developed at the site of infusion in only 1 of the 22 patients who received the drug intravenously.

Comment

In vitro, cephapirin was very effective in inhibiting growth of gram-positive cocci except enterococci. *E. coli*, *Klebsiella* and *Proteus mirabilis* required greater concentrations of cephapirin for growth inhibition in brain-heart infusion broth than most gram-positive cocci. All strains of *Pseudomonas aeruginosa* and most of *Enterobacter* appeared to be highly resistant to this drug.

The geometric mean MIC of our strains of *E. coli* and *Proteus mirabilis* was significantly lower in nutrient broth than in brain-heart infusion broth. This may explain why the MIC's of cephapirin for strains of *E. coli* and *Proteus mirabilis* in our study were somewhat higher than those determined by some investigators.[7]

The MIC's of most strains of *E. coli*, *Klebsiella* and *Proteus mirabilis* were in a range of drug concentrations that could readily be achieved in the urine of patients with normal renal function. However, when considered in terms of serum concentrations achievable with the usual dosage regimens, bacteremia caused by some of those gram-negative bacilli might not be expected to respond to cephapirin. This was evident in one of our patients who had endocarditis due to a strain of *E. coli* requiring 50 μg/ml of cephapirin for growth inhibition. Bacteremia persisted despite 12 gm of cephapirin given intravenously daily for

Infection	Causative Organism (M I C of cephapirin μg/ml)	Result of Treatment
Wound infection	*E. coli (7100)* and *Proteus mirabilis* (25)	Qualified success*
	Staphylococcus aureus (0.1)	Qualified success*
Chronic osteo-myelitis	*Proteus mirabilis* (12.5)	Qualified success*
Septic arthritis	*Staphylococcus aureus* (0.2)	Qualified success*

*Lesion healed but post-treatment cultures were not obtained because there was no drainage material to culture.

TABLE 6

Results of Cephapirin Therapy in 4 Patients with Miscellaneous Infections

several days; subsequently the bloodstream infection was eradicated with ampicillin (MIC = 4 μg/ml).

In general, cephapirin appeared to be effective for treatment of serious infections caused by susceptible organisms in patients who did not have underlying noninfectious diseases that precluded recovery. There was a low incidence of pain or phlebitis at sites of injection and no evidence of nephrotoxicity. The relatively high incidence of allergic reactions in our patients warrants further study. Since cephapirin is rapidly excreted in patients with

TABLE 7

Adverse Effects of Cephapirin*

	Number of Patients
Elevated SGOT	5
Eosinophilia	4
Drug fever	3
Elevated serum alkaline phosphatase	2
Leukopenia	1
Phlebitis	1
Generalized maculopapular rash	1
Bullous erythema multiforme	1
TOTAL	9**

*One patient with hemolytic anemia of multipotential etiology not included in table.

**More than one side effect was noted in several patients.

normal renal function, parenteral doses should be given at intervals of at least every four to six hours. Dosage regimens of cephapirin for patients with impaired renal function require further study.

Summary

Two hundred ninety strains of gram-positive cocci and gram-negative bacilli were tested for susceptibility *in vitro* against cephapirin. The drug was highly effective in inhibiting growth of gram-positive cocci except enterococci. It was somewhat less effective against gram-negative bacilli. The mean serum half-life of cephapirin in persons with normal renal function was 0.6 hr. Cephapirin appeared to be effective for treatment of serious infections caused by susceptible organisms. There was a low incidence of pain or phlebitis at sites of injection and no evidence of nephrotoxicity. The relatively high incidence of allergic reactions warrants further study.

REFERENCES

1. Chisholm DR, Leitner F, Wright GE, et al: Laboratory studies with a new cephalosporanic acid derivative. Antimicrobial Agents and Chemotherapy — 1969, 1970 American Society for Microbiology, pp 244-246.
2. Gordon RC, Barrett FF, Clark DJ et al: Laboratory and pharmacologic studies of BL-P-1322 (cephapirin sodium) in children. Curr Ther Research 13:398-406, 1971.
3. Cephapirin Sodium (BL-P-1322) Basic Data Brochure, Department of Medical Research, Bristol Laboratories, Syracuse, New York.
4. Gavan TL: Bacteriology. Manual of Clinical Laboratory Procedures, 2nd Edition, Faulkner WR and King JW ed, Cleveland, Ohio, The Chemical Rubber Company, 1970, pp 249-311.
5. Gavan TL and Town MA: A microdilution method for antibiotic susceptibility testing: An evaluation. Am J Clin Pathol 53:880-885, 1970.
6. Bauer WA, Kirby WMM, Sherris JC, et al: Antibiotic susceptibility testing by a standardized single disc method. Am J Clin Pathol 45:493-496, 1966.
7. Turck M: Personal communication.

PARENTERAL CLINDAMYCIN IN THE TREATMENT OF INFECTIONS

• A preliminary clinical study in a limited number of patients suggest that parenteral clindamycin is an effective well-tolerated agent in the treatment of gram-positive coccal infections.

CHRISTOPHER ROYER DONOHO, JR., M.D.

Clindamycin* (7-chloro-7-deoxylincomycin) is a lincomycin analogue and like the parent drug, has a narrow spectrum of effectiveness *in vitro* and *in vivo* against the gram-positive cocci, excluding the enterococci. Clindamycin and lincomycin are both small molecules with less potential for sensitization than the penicillin-type antibiotics and therefore may be useful in patients with a history of penicillin allergy or multiple drug sensitivities.

Clindamycin appears to be more effective *in vitro* than lincomycin, allowing a lower dosage of this analogue for clinical efficacy. The reported lower incidence of gastrointestinal side effects with clindamycin therapy may be the result of this lower dosage requirement.[1-3]

The oral preparation of clindamycin is available for clinical use in the United States, and there are a number of reports in the literature concerning its efficacy.[1-3] The parenteral form of clindamycin is available only for investigational use and less information is available concerning clinical experience with this preparation. This preliminary report records the experience in a study designed to evaluate the clinical efficacy of parenteral clindamycin in the treatment of infections due to gram-positive cocci (excluding enterococci).

Material and Methods

Twenty-one patients from the Medical and Surgical Services were selected for inclusion in the study. Thirteen of the patients were male, and eight were female, their ages rang-

ing from 19 to 74. Several of the patients had a previous history of penicillin sensitivity, and all twenty-one patients were suffering from pneumonia and/or infections of the bone or soft tissue.

The antibiotic was supplied by the Upjohn Company as clindamycin-2-phosphate in 2 ml vials each containing 300 mg. The intravenous dose was 300 to 450 mg given by a rapid drip (30 minutes) every eight hours, while the intramuscular dose was 300 mg every eight to twelve hours. The duration of parenteral therapy usually ranged from two to twelve days though one patient with streptococcal osteomyelitis received the parenteral antibiotic for twenty-six days. In two patients the clindamycin-2-phosphate was first administered intravenously with a subsequent change to the intramuscular route.

Pre-and post-treatment cultures were obtained on all patients treated with clindamycin, and pre- and post-treatment hemograms, chemistry 12 profiles and urinalyses were obtained in most instances.

Results

Table 1 details the clinical data in seventeen of the twenty-one patients who had clinical evidence of bacterial pneumonia. Despite the clinical profile of bacterial pneumonia, ten of the original sputum cultures in these seventeen patients revealed only normal flora. In three patients the sputum culture revealed a pneumococcus and in an additional two patients, the cultures yielded pneumococcus and *Hemophilus influenzae*. In one patient, the original sputum culture grew a *Proteus* species. One of the seventeen patients showed no pathogen in the sputum culture

*Cleocin® Upjohn Company, Kalamazoo, Michigan

Dr. Donoho is a Resident in Internal Medicine, Wilmington Medical Center.

185

TABLE 1

PNEUMONIA PATIENTS TREATED WITH PARENTERAL CLINDAMYCIN

Number of Patients	ORGANISM	TREATMENT	RESPONSE
3	No pathogen	300-600 Q8h I.V. four-twelve days	Success
1	Pneumococcus	450 Q8h I.V. four days 600 Q12h six days	Success
1	Group A strep. blood	450 Q8h I.V. two days medication changed	Success
7	No pathogen	300 Q12h IM four-twelve days	Success
2	Pneumococcus	300 Q12h IM seven-eleven days	Success
2	Pneumococcus *H. influenzae*	300 Q12h IM nine-twelve days	Success
1	*Proteus* species	300 Q12h IM two days	Failure

though the blood culture grew a beta-hemolytic streptococcus (group A). Except for the one patient whose initial sputum culture revealed a *Proteus* species, all the pneumonia patients showed a satisfactory clinical response following parenteral clindamycin therapy given for two to twelve days. A satisfactory response is defined here as rapid (that is, eight to twelve hours) defervescence of fever, decrease of chest pain and malaise, and evidence of radiologic clearing of the area of infiltration.

Table 2 details the results of clindamycin therapy in six patients with infections of bone and/or soft tissues. Two of these six patients also suffered from pneumonia and were reported on the previous table. All six patients with soft tissue or bone infection showed a satisfactory response to parenteral clindamycin therapy. Two patients with osteomyelitis (in one instance due to beta-hemolytic streptococcus and the other to *Staphylococcus aureus*) experienced a successful outcome after twenty-six days' and ten days' therapy, respectively. Likewise, the patient with the eye infection due to coagulase-negative staphylococcus and the patient with *Staphylococcus aureus* infection of an ankle cutdown site, both showed a successful response to clindamycin therapy. A patient with sacral cellulitis due to a coagulase-positive *Staphylococcus aureus* and a beta-hemolytic streptococcus, responded to ten days of therapy with parenteral clindamycin. More difficult to evaluate was a patient with scrotal cellulitis with a multiplicity of microorganisms isolated from the wound surface. Four days of parenteral clindamycin followed by oral clindamycin therapy resulted in a satisfactory, though slow, response. Parenteral clindamycin therapy was successful in eliminating the pathogens from these bone and soft tissue lesions in each instance.

Side Effects

There were no untoward reactions to clindamycin in the twenty-one patients included in this study. No gastrointestinal disturbance or undue irritation at the site of administration was reported. There was no significant alteration in the hemogram, chemistry 12 profile or urinalysis in any of these patients. Four patients who received intramuscular clindamycin had significant elevations of creatinine phosphokinase with slight eleva-

TABLE 2

BONE AND SOFT TISSUE INFECTIONS TREATED WITH PARENTERAL CLINDAMYCIN

Diagnosis	Organism	Treatment	Response
Wound infection in ankle cutdown	*Staphylococcus aureus* Coagulase-positive	300 mg IM Q12h for eleven days	Success
Scrotal cellulitis	*Escherichia coli* *Enterobacter* Enterococcus *Bacteroides* Peptostreptococcus	300 mg IM Q12h for four days	Success
Eye infection*	Coagulase-negative Staphylococcus Group D strep.	450 mg I.V. Q8h for two days then medication changed	Success
Osteomyelitis**	Beta-hemolytic Strep. (not D)	300 mg IM Q12h for twenty-six days	Success
Osteomyelitis	*Staphylococcus aureus* Coagulase-negative	300 mg IM Q12h for ten days	Success
Sacral cellulitis*	*Staphylococcus aureus* Coagulase-positive Beta-hemolytic Strep.	300 mg IM Q12h for ten days	Success

*Patients also reported on in Table 1.
**Patient expired from acute myocardial infarction while on therapy.

tions of the serum glutamic oxaloacetic trans-aminase but no elevation in the liver enzymes. It was assumed that these abnormalities were due to the intramuscular administration of clindamycin.

In two instances, superinfection occurred while patients were receiving clindamycin therapy. One patient developed an enter-ococcal urinary tract infection, complicating bladder drainage with an indwelling bladder catheter while receiving I.V. clindamycin therapy. The second patient, also with an in-dwelling bladder catheter, developed a *Serratia* urinary tract infection while receiving intramuscular clindamycin. Both patients were subsequently successfully treated with an appropriate antibiotic.

Summary

This study was not designed to compare the effectiveness of clindamycin with the parent antibiotic lincomycin or other currently available antibiotics, but rather to afford clinical experience in the treatment of infections with the parenteral form of clindamycin. This new antibiotic appears to be similar to the parent compound in spectrum, efficacy, tolerance and toxicity. Twenty-one patients suspected of having gram-positive infections were treated with clindamycin with a satisfactory response in each instance except for a patient with bacterial pneumonia apparently due to *Proteus* species.

There were no significant gastrointestinal side effects with the absence of diarrhea being particularly noteworthy.

REFERENCES

1. Hogan LB and Holloway WJ: An evaluation of 7-chlorolincomy-cin. Presented at the Eighth Interscience on Antimicrobial Agents and Chemotherapy. New York, New York, October 1968.
2. Holloway WJ: Lincomycin and clindamycin in the treatment of severe infections. Presented at the Sixth International Congress of Chemotherapy. Tokyo, Japan, August 1969.
3. Oppenheimer S and Turck M: Laboratory and clinical evaluation of 7-chloro-7-deoxylincomycin: Amer J Med Sci 256:314-320, 1968.

PRELIMINARY REPORT

ON INTRAVENOUS DOXYCYCLINE

• Tetracycline derivatives that do not depend upon renal excretion for elimination from the body should have less potential for accumulation in the body and production of the catabolic tetracycline side effects.

WILLIAM J. HOLLOWAY, M.D.

Doxycycline, the newest of the oral tetracyclines to be available for clinical use in the United States, differs from the older tetracyclines in several pharmacokinetic properties. This antibiotic appears to be rapidly and almost completely absorbed from the gastrointestinal tract, and a slow elimination rate results in a half life of about twenty hours. The renal clearance of doxycycline is about 23 ml per minute, this being significantly less than the other tetracycline compounds. Apparently the liver is responsible for most of the clearance of doxycycline from the body.

This new tetracycline has been used successfully in the treatment of acute and chronic urinary tract infections,[1,2] being effective in a once daily dosage because of the prolonged half life and excellent blood levels after oral absorption. The reported[1,2] low incidence of side effects from doxycycline may be due in part to the lower total dose of tetracycline administered to the patient.

There is limited evidence[2] that doxycycline is more effective in vitro against certain strains of Pseudomonas aeruginosa, and patients with chronic Pseudomonas urinary tract infection have been controlled with long-term doxycycline therapy after failing to respond to other antibacterial agents.[2]

Tetracycline's catabolic effect on cells, mediated through its interference with the absorption of essential amino acids,[3,4] has limited the use of this antibiotic in patients who are critically ill with concurrent impairment of kidney and liver function. Klinger and his coworkers[5] have suggested that doxycycline might be given safely to patients with renal insufficiency because drug accumulation and cumulative toxicity are not to be expected. Additional clinical experience is necessary to further substantiate this hypothesis. This paper is a preliminary report on the clinical trial of an intravenous formulation of doxycycline.

Material and Methods

Patients on the Medical and Surgical Services of the Wilmington Medical Center in whom tetracycline appeared to be the antibiotic of choice were considered as candidates for inclusion in this study. Since this tetracycline was to be administered by the intravenous route, an additional prerequisite was that the patient require parenteral administration of antibiotic because of the inability to swallow or tolerate oral medication.

The intravenous preparation of doxycycline* was supplied by Charles Pfizer and Company in a powder form and was dissolved in 500 to 1000 ml of diluent (5% glucose and water or normal saline solution) for intravenous administration. Patients treated early in the study were given 100 mg of doxycycline dissolved in 500 ml of diluent as a drip over four to six hours. Because of local irritation (to be described later in the paper) subsequent patients were given doxycycline 100 mg

Dr. Holloway is Director, Infectious Disease Research Laboratory, Wilmington Medical Center, Wilmington, Delaware.

* Vibramycin®

dissolved in 1000 ml of diluent administered over a period of eight to twelve hours. The intravenous doxycycline was administered for a minimum of three days in all patients and in some patients as long as nine days (mean duration of intravenous doxycycline therapy equals four days). In all but two patients the intravenous doxycycline was followed by a course of oral doxycycline therapy.

Pre- and post-treatment cultures were taken on all patients included in the study, and the pathogens isolated were tested for doxycycline susceptibility by the agar-disc diffusion technique and in some instances by the test-tube dilution technique. When feasible, follow-up cultures were done on the day intravenous doxycycline therapy was discontinued as well as at the completion of all antibiotic therapy. Other laboratory parameters measured before and after doxycycline therapy included complete blood count with platelet count, chemistry 12 profile and urinalysis. In instances where there was an elevation of the blood urea nitrogen, the serum creatinine was also measured serially. A total of 22 patients have now been treated with this intravenous formulation of doxycycline.

Results

Table 1 details the type of infection present in the twenty-two patients treated with intravenous doxycycline and the results of therapy. Fourteen patients with urinary tract infection received this antibiotic with ten patients experiencing a successful outcome. One patient failed to respond to therapy, and three patients were characterized as having an indeterminate response. Eleven of the fourteen patients were considered to have acute urinary tract infection while two patients were classified as chronic. In one patient there was a history of recurrent infection.

The patient who failed to respond to tetracycline therapy was a 34-year-old female patient with end stage renal disease and chronic pyelonephritis who failed to respond to therapy with several other antibiotics prior to the administration of intravenous doxycycline.

One patient with an indeterminate result was a 33-year-old female patient who had acute pyelonephritis associated with peritonitis and pneumonia. Bacteriuria (*Escherichia coli* and *Pseudomonas aeruginosa*) was eradicated by doxycycline therapy, but the fever did not defervesce during her course of therapy.

The second patient with an indeterminate response to intravenous doxycycline was a male patient with Reiter's Syndrome, the urethritis apparently due to mycoplasma T-strain. While he showed significant improvement during intravenous doxycycline therapy, his response was slow, and complete clearing required ten days of oral doxycycline therapy.

An additional indeterminate response was in a patient in whom doxycycline therapy was instituted when bacterial infection complicating an indwelling Foley catheter was suspected. The patient improved on intravenous doxycycline therapy, but initial cultures of the urine were negative. The indwelling catheter was subsequently removed, and a culture of the catheter tip revealed a significant growth of *Staphylococcus aureus*, tetracycline sensitive. While this patient appeared to have a satisfactory response on doxycycline therapy, the absence of a positive culture prior to the institution of therapy precludes conclusive evaluation.

Six of the twenty-two patients included in this study were treated for bacterial pneumonia, and all six patients responded to therapy. In three instances the infecting microorganism was *H. influenza*, and in one instance each, the primary pathogen was beta streptococcus, pneumococcus and *Mycoplasma pneumoniae*.

A patient with septicemia due to *Klebsiella* type 35 failed to respond to intravenous doxycycline therapy. This patient was in a terminal stage of leukemia and had failed to respond to numerous other antibiotic agents prior to a trial with this antibiotic.

The final patient in this study was a twenty-six-year-old female with gonococcal cervicitis, urethritis, and pyarthrosis who showed a favorable clinical response to three days of intravenous doxycycline therapy and negative cultures at the time oral doxycycline therapy

Type of Infection	Number of Cases	Success	Failure	Indeterminate
URINARY TRACT	14	10	1	3
PNEUMONIA	6	6	0	0
SEPTICEMIA (*Klebsiella* type 35)	1	0	1	0
GONOCOCCAL Cervicitis-Pyarthrosis	1	1	0	0

TABLE 1

RESULTS OF THERAPY
INTRAVENOUS DOXYCYCLINE

was substituted for the parenteral preparation.

Side Effects and Toxicity

Significant local phlebitis with severe pain occurred in five patients receiving intravenous doxycycline therapy in this study. In all five of the patients, the phlebitis necessitated frequent changing of the intravenous catheter site, and in one patient it was necessary to discontinue intravenous doxycycline therapy on the third day because of severe distress. It should be noted that all five of the patients who experienced significant local irritation from the intravenous doxycycline were receiving 100 mg of the antibiotic dissolved in 500 ml of diluent. The remaining patients who received their doxycycline in 1000 ml of diluent did not complain of significant local irritation and experienced an incidence of local phlebitis comparable to that seen in our institution in patients receiving any type of intravenous therapy.

Five patients in this study group had a significant elevation of blood urea nitrogen at the time intravenous doxycycline therapy was instituted. All of these patients tolerated the intravenous doxycycline therapy well and did not show any significant elevation of blood urea nitrogen during therapy. In fact, four of the five patients experienced a significant decrease in the blood urea nitrogen level during the period of administration of the intravenous antibiotic.

In one patient there was a significant increase in the blood urea nitrogen level during doxycycline therapy. This was a 54-year-old-female patient with diabetes mellitus and congestive heart failure who required an indwelling bladder catheter on admission to the hospital and subsequently developed a symptomatic urinary tract infection due to a *Klebsiella* species and an enterococcus. The catheter was removed and intravenous doxycycline therapy instituted. At this time the blood urea nitrogen was 33 mg/100 ml, the serum creatinine was 2 mg/100 ml and a creatinine clearance was 15.3 ml/min. Intravenous doxycycline in a dosage of 100 mg twice daily was continued for a five-day period, and the patient was subsequently placed on oral doxycycline in the same dosage. Because of a technical error, the blood urea nitrogen was not determined until two days after intravenous doxycycline was discontinued. At this time the blood urea nitrogen was 123 mg/100 ml, and the serum creatinine 3 mg/100 ml. The oral doxycycline was discontinued on the following day, and blood urea nitrogen determinations done daily revealed an elevated level for an additional week. Eleven days after cessation of doxycycline therapy, the blood urea nitrogen was 16 mg/100 ml and the serum creatinine 1.5 mg/100 ml. It is conceivable that this occurrence represents an instance of the uremic syndrome occurring in a patient on doxycycline therapy. However, the attending physician responsible for this patient was of the opinion that untimely removal of the indwelling bladder catheter as well as dehydration may have been contributing factors in the elevation of the blood urea nitrogen. It should be noted that there was a minimal increase in the serum creatinine level during the uremic period.

191

Summary

Doxycycline, the newest tetracycline antibiotic, has a low renal clearance in normal individuals, suggesting that it may have less potential toxicity in critically ill patients with impaired renal function.

This preliminary clinical report on intravenous doxycycline records satisfactory results in ten of fourteen patients with urinary tract infection and all six patients with bacterial pneumonia. A patient with terminal leukemia and *Klebsiella* type 35 septicemia failed to respond to the antibiotic, while a patient with gonococcal pyarthrosis complicating cervicitis and urethritis did respond to intravenous doxycycline therapy.

Local phlebitis with severe burning discomfort at the injection site was common in patients who received the 100 mg dose of doxycycline dissolved in only 500 ml of diluent. When the quantity of diluent was increased to 1000 ml, this local irritation no longer occurred.

Five patients with significant elevation of the blood urea nitrogen at the time intravenous doxycycline therapy was instituted showed no evidence of doxcycline toxicity. A fifty-four-year-old diabetic with pyelonephritis and pulmonary edema had slight elevation of the blood urea nitrogen and serum creatinine at the time therapy with doxycycline was instituted. During subsequent therapy with the intravenous and oral preparation of the antibiotic, there was a marked rise in blood urea nitrogen with a slight rise in serum creatinine. After cessation of therapy, these parameters slowly returned to normal. Factors other than doxycycline therapy may have been responsible for these altered laboratory values.

Further clinical trial of intravenous doxycycline seems warranted and is underway at the Wilmington Medical Center.

REFERENCES

1. Colmore JP, Braden B and Wilkerson R: Effectiveness of doxycycline treatment in chronic urinary tract infections. Antimicrobial Agents and Chemotherapy, 1966, p 118.
2: Holloway WJ, Furlong JH and Scott EG: Doxycycline in the treatment of infections of the urinary tract. Journ of Urology 102:249-252, 1969.
3. Shils ME: Renal disease and the metabolic effects of tetracycline. Annals of Intern Med 58:389-413, 1963.
4. Faloon WW, Downs JJ, Duggan K et al: Nitrogen and electrolyte metabolism and hepatic function and histology in patients receiving tetracycline. Amer Journ Med Scien 233:563-572, 1957.
5. Klinger W, Bayerl P and Edel H: Doxycycline in renal insufficiency. Progress in Antimicrobial and Anticancer Chemotherapy (Proceedings of the 6th International Congress of Chemotherapy) 1:605-608, 1970.

I do not forget that Medicine and Veterinary practice are foreign to me. I desire judgment and' criticism upon all my contributions. Little tolerant of frivolous or prejudiced contradiction, contemptuous of that ignorant criticism which doubts on principle, I welcome with open arms the militant attack which has a method in doubting and whose rule of conduct has the motto "More light."
The Germ Theory and Its Applications to Medicine and Surgery, Ch. 12,